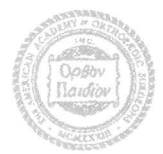

American Academy of Orthopaedic
6300 North River Road
Rosemont, Illinois 60018
1-800-626-6726

# Chronic Ankle Pain in the Athlete

**EDITED BY**
**GLENN B. PFEFFER, MD**
Assistant Clinical Professor
Department of Orthopaedics
University of California, San Francisco
San Francisco, California

**CONTRIBUTORS**
Richard D. Ferkel, MD
Carol Frey, MD
Vincent James Sammarco, MD
Lew C. Schon, MD
Pierce E. Scranton, Jr, MD

**SERIES EDITOR**
Thomas R. Johnson, MD

Director, Department of Publications
*Marilyn L. Fox, PhD*

Managing Editor
*Lynne Roby Shindoll*

Production Manager
*Loraine Edwalds*

Assistant Production Manager
*Sophie Tosta*

Graphic Design Coordinator
*Pamela Hutton Erickson*

Editorial Assistant
*Anu Amaran*

Production Assistants
*Geraldine Dubberke*
*Jana Ronayne*
*Vanessa Villarreal*

Publications Secretary
*Jackie Shadinger*

**Board of Directors 1999**

*Robert D. D'Ambrosia, MD*
President

*S. Terry Canale, MD*
First Vice President

*Richard H. Gelberman, MD*
Second Vice President

*William J. Robb III, MD*
Secretary

*Stuart A. Hirsch, MD*
Treasurer

*David A. Halsey, MD*
*James D. Heckman, MD*
*Joseph P. Iannotti, MD*
*Douglas W. Jackson, MD*
*Ramon L. Jimenez, MD*
*Thomas P. Schmalzried, MD*
*William A. Sims, MD*
*Vernon T. Tolo, MD*
*John R. Tongue, MD*
*Edward A. Toriello, MD*
*Richard B. Welch, MD*
*William W. Tipton, Jr, MD (Ex Officio)*

The American Academy of Orthopaedic Surgeons Monograph Series is dedicated to Wendy O. Schmidt, American Academy of Orthopaedic Surgeons senior medical editor, 1987-1991.

## CHRONIC ANKLE PAIN IN THE ATHLETE
American Academy of Orthopaedic Surgeons®

The material presented in *Chronic Ankle Pain in the Athlete* has been made available by the American Academy of Orthopaedic Surgeons® for educational purposes only. This material is not intended to present the only, or necessarily best, methods or procedures for the medical situations discussed, but rather is intended to represent an approach, view, statement, or opinion of the author(s) or producer(s), which may be helpful to others who face similar situations.

Some drugs or medical devices demonstrated in Academy print or electronic publications have not been cleared by the Food and Drug Administration (FDA) or have been cleared by the FDA for specific uses only. The FDA has stated that it is the responsibility of the physician to determine the FDA clearance status of each drug or device he or she wishes to use in clinical practice.

Furthermore, any statements about commercial products are solely the opinion of the author(s) and do not represent an Academy endorsement or evaluation of these products. These statements may not be used in advertising or for any commercial purpose.

All rights reserved. No part of this publication may be reproduced, stored in a retrieval system, or transmitted, in any form, or by any means, electronic, mechanical, photocopying, recording, or otherwise, without prior written permission from the publisher.

First Edition
Copyright © 2000 by the
American Academy of Orthopaedic Surgeons®

ISBN 0-89203-226-X

# CONTENTS

| | |
|---|---|
| **PREFACE** | vii |
| **INTRODUCTION** | 1 |
| **SPRAINS AND SOFT-TISSUE INJURIES** | 3 |
| **INJURIES TO THE SUBTALAR JOINT** | 21 |
| **ARTHROSCOPIC TREATMENT OF OSTEOCHONDRAL LESIONS, SOFT-TISSUE IMPINGEMENT, AND LOOSE BODIES** | 43 |
| **NERVE INJURIES OF THE LATERAL LEG AND ANKLE** | 71 |
| **INDEX** | 85 |

# CONTRIBUTORS

Richard D. Ferkel, MD
Attending Surgeon and Fellowship Director
Southern California Orthopedic Institute
Van Nuys, California

Carol Frey, MD
Interim Clinical Professor
Department of Orthopaedic Surgery
University of California, Los Angeles
Manhattan Beach, California

Vincent James Sammarco, MD
The Center for Orthopaedic Care
Cincinnati, Ohio

Lew C. Schon, MD
Assistant Director, Foot and Ankle Services
Department of Orthopaedic Surgery
The Union Memorial Hospital
Baltimore, Maryland

Pierce E. Scranton, Jr, MD
Orthopedic Surgeon
Orthopedics International, LTD P.S.
Seattle, Washington

## PREFACE

An ankle sprain is one of the most common injuries associated with sports participation. While most athletes return to full activity, up to 40% experience chronic symptoms. Invariably, these symptoms involve the lateral and anterolateral aspects of the ankle. Unfortunately, the diagnosis "chronic ankle sprain" is still often used to explain persistent symptoms, even though inadequate rehabilitation or missed pathology is the true cause. The focus of this monograph is the evaluation and treatment of the common, as well as often overlooked, causes of chronic lateral and anterolateral ankle pain: occult fracture, cartilage injury, ankle and subtalar instability, soft-tissue impingement, peroneal tendon pathology, and nerve entrapment.

I have been fortunate to work with an outstanding group of authors who are experts in the field of foot and ankle care. They and their staffs have worked tirelessly to produce an outstanding monograph. The staff of the Academy Publications Department should also be acknowledged, as they worked diligently to keep the monograph moving through all phases of development and production.

**GLENN B. PFEFFER, MD**

# INTRODUCTION

## GLEN B. PFEFFER, MD

Nine million Americans sprain their ankles every year, and of these, more than 2 million are left with chronic symptoms. Athletes, especially those who participate in running and jumping sports, experience the highest incidence of chronic symptoms. The most common of these include intermittent stiffness, swelling, weakness, giving way, and pain. Chronic medial symptoms can occur but are rare. Posterior tibial tendon pathology is the most common cause of chronic medial pain, and in the athlete, is usually related to a chronic tendinitis from overuse. The preponderance of chronic symptoms, however, affect the anterior and anterolateral aspects of the ankle and are the focus of this monograph.

Athletes typically present with a history of intermittent symptoms that have persisted for 6 months or longer. Most can trace the onset of their symptoms to a previous moderate to severe ankle sprain, although insidious onset is not uncommon. Many athletes will have already received some manner of treatment and are now seeking a second opinion, frustrated with persistent symptoms and the delay in return to activity.

The initial clinical history should include the following questions:

1. ***Has the athlete had a previous significant ankle sprain?*** More than half of the athletes who have sprained an ankle will sprain it again. The most common predisposing factor for an ankle sprain is having had sprained the same ankle in the past.

2. ***Does the athlete report constant pain?*** Constant pain, no matter how mild, is diagnostic of certain conditions, such as occult fracture, posttraumatic arthritis, peroneal tendon tear, or, rarely, complex regional pain syndrome (CRPS).

3. ***Is there a history of repeated sprains or flare-ups with the athlete asymptomatic between episodes?*** Conditions such as ankle or subtalar instability or intermittent peroneal tendon dislocation are consistent with this history.

4. ***In athletes with repeated sprains, does the sprain precede or follow the onset of pain?*** An episode of giving way is often precipitated by the acute onset of pain. An osteochondral lesion of the talus (OLT) or an intra-articular loose body are common causes of acute pain that can cause an athlete to misstep and experience a sprain.

5. ***Does the athlete report pain with specific activities, such as hill running, equinus sports, or traversing uneven ground?*** A history of these symptoms is consistent with diagnoses of anterior impingement, posterior impingement, or subtalar dysfunction, respectively.

6. ***How soon did the athlete return to sports following a sprain?*** Many athletes resume activity prematurely without adequate rehabilitation. Symptoms that persist 4 to 5 months after an initial injury may require nothing more than an intensive course of rehabilitation or physical therapy that emphasizes Achilles tendon stretching, ankle and subtalar range of motion, strength training, and proprioception training. The latter is probably the most important factor in return to full activity, but is the one area of rehabilitation that is most often overlooked. Use of ankle tape or a brace should be encouraged upon return to activity to avoid recurrent sprains and possible permanent injury.

After the history is obtained, careful clinical examination is needed to confirm the diagnosis. Athletes are often unable to localize their symptoms by history, and focal tenderness on examination is the key to the correct diagnosis. For example, focal tenderness at the site of a peroneal tendon tear, nerve entrapment, lateral gutter impingement, or sinus tarsi syndrome is easy to elicit with one-finger palpation. Focal tenderness is also present over a malunion or nonunion of an occult fracture (eg, anterolateral, posterolateral, or lateral process of the calcaneus, OLT, base of the fifth metatarsal, stress fracture of the fibula). Varus or anterior instability should be evident on examination and can be confirmed by stress radiographs. Painful or decreased subtalar motion is consistent with the following diagnoses: posttraumatic arthritis, tarsal coalition, or soft-tissue impingements of the subtalar joint. Subtalar motion may be difficult to evaluate, however, as abnormal varus laxity of the ankle joint can be mistaken for normal motion of the subtalar joint. Subtalar pathology is perhaps the most commonly missed of all chronic conditions of the foot and ankle; therefore, this part of the examination requires special attention.

CRPS is typically a straightforward diagnosis. Early presentation, characterized by disproportionate pain, increased warmth, and venous distention of the involved extremity, is often under diagnosed. However, in athletes with chronic pain, CRPS is often over diagnosed. The multiple causes of chronic ankle symptoms must always be excluded before the diagnosis of CRPS is made.

Advanced imaging techniques play an important role in the evaluation of chronic ankle pain. Intra-articular lesions of the ankle and subtalar joint may be especially difficult to diagnose by history and clinical examination alone. Technetium 99m bone scans are invaluable in screening for occult osseous injuries and should be obtained early in the work-up of athletes with chronic ankle pain. Normal results on clinical examination in conjunction with a normal bone scan essentially excludes all causes of chronic pain except soft-tissue impingements.

MRI and CT are of little use in the screening process. Both studies should be reserved for evaluating specific diagnoses and in preoperative planning. In most instances, CT is indicated to evaluate a focal abnormality seen on a bone scan. MRI is appropriate for evaluating soft-tissue pathology detected on examination. The imaging study most appropriate for evaluating osteochondral lesions remains controversial. Although CT is preferred by some authors, new MRI techniques provide information about the overlying articular cartilage, which is invaluable for surgical planning.

Normal bone scans, MRI, and CT scans do not exclude all causes of chronic pain. Soft-tissue impingement of the ankle or subtalar joint and a relatively small percentage of peroneal tendon tears will not be detected by these studies. In these athletes, differential injection with lidocaine plays an essential role in making the correct diagnosis. Differential injections will also help confirm that an abnormal finding on an imaging study is the actual source of an athlete's symptoms. These issues are discussed in greater detail in the chapters that follow.

In summary, chronic pain in the anterior and anterolateral aspects of the ankle in athletes is a common problem with uncommon causes. Incomplete rehabilitation is one important cause, but other possibilities must be considered and evaluated. Symptoms that persist for 4 months following an ankle sprain require evaluation for possible additional rehabilitation. At this juncture, if careful clinical examination and technetium 99m bone scans are normal, then a formal course of physical therapy and sport-specific rehabilitation is likely to be sufficient. Abnormalities on examination or on bone scan require further evaluation by MRI or CT. Differential lidocaine injections are also very helpful. Ultimately, surgical intervention may be required so that the athlete can return to full participation and performance.

# SPRAINS AND SOFT-TISSUE INJURIES

PIERCE E. SCRANTON, JR, MD

## INTRODUCTION

An estimated 27,000 ankle sprains occur each day in the United States. The true number is unknown because a significant percentage of patients do not seek medical care. The spectrum of injuries is significant. In this section I will focus on nonsurgical and surgical management in 3 specific areas: ankle sprains, syndesmosis injuries, and peroneal tendon injuries.

## ANKLE SPRAINS

### DEFINITION

An ankle sprain can be broadly defined as a soft-tissue injury that occurs when the motion of the talus within the mortise exceeds the physiologic limits imposed by the restraining ligaments. Depending on the direction(s) of translation and forces applied, the injury or sprain is defined as a grade I, II, or III injury. The deltoid, anterior talofibular (ATF), calcaneofibular (CFL), or posterior talofibular (PTF) ligaments are singularly, or in combination capable of sustaining a sprain.

### GRADING

For purposes of simplicity, a grading system with grades I to III has been adopted to describe the severity of the injury. The grade of sprain does not apply to associated pathology that can often cause the greatest morbidity. Furthermore, it represents a debated area of esoteric semantics, because grades I and II represent partial sprain of one or more ligaments, whereas a grade III sprain is actually ligamentous disruption of one or more ankle ligaments.

### Grade I

A grade I sprain is an injury in which the ankle ligament has retained its stability, but there has been some interstitial disruption of fibers. Patients presenting with a grade I sprain usually are able to walk, placing weight on the involved limb. Discrete tenderness occurs only at the site of the ligament injury, with localized minimal swelling. Because the magnitude of injury-producing force is low, generally only one ligament is involved. There usually is no associated pathology.

### Grade II

A grade II sprain is more complex. More force has been applied, partially disrupting one or more ligaments. Patients presenting with a grade II sprain may or may not be able to bear weight on the affected ankle. The ankle swelling and pain are more diffuse, indicating that significant bleeding from one or both partially torn ligaments is present. A careful comparison of the involved ankle to the uninvolved ankle often reveals asymmetric stability. The ligament is still functional but the fibers have been damaged such that, with stress, the talus could sublux within the mortise. With grade II injuries, the physician should consider the likelihood of associated articular or periarticular pathology.

### Grade III

A grade III sprain involves a complete disruption of at least one ligament. Most patients who have a grade III sprain are unable to walk. The swelling is significant and a hemarthrosis of the ankle joint usually is present. The entire medial and lateral ankle are swollen such that relaxation of the spasmed peroneal tendons is difficult at best. These evertors protectively spasm to support the ankle. The hemarthrosis distends the joint capsule so that the ankle is held in a plantarflexed position for greater comfort. Dorsiflexion is painful. Some physicians have advocated examination under anesthesia for the better assessment of stability. Subjecting the patient to anesthetic risks merely to confirm a major obvious ligament disruption seems unnecessary. If the patient can relax the foot and ankle enough in plantarflexion, a stress test will reveal significant anterior and/or varus talar instability with no end point. In a grade III disruption, the possibility of associated intra-articular or periarticular injury is high.

## ASSOCIATED PATHOLOGY

Pathology associated with ankle sprains is described extensively in appropriate sections of this chapter. The reasons for this pathology are briefly described here. For example, in a grade III ligament disruption it is helpful for the clinician to think of the ankle simplistically, as though it were a ring: if one side is broken, the other side has to break too. Another example works according to Newton's second law, "for every action there is an equal and opposite reaction." In an isolated, severe, inversion injury with the ankle in neutral flexion, the calcaneofibular ligament tears as the talus inverts. At the same time, the medial dome of the talus strikes the tibial plafond and an osteochondral injury can occur. If three-dimensional forces are added to this circumstance, the possibilities for associated articular and periarticular pathology are extensive.

## DIAGNOSTIC MEASURES

Patient history is important in ascertaining the severity of the injury and the structures injured. A key determinant of the course of treatment is whether this is the first injury to this ankle. The next determinant is the exact mechanism of injury. Did the athlete experience a "pop" or snap in the ankle? Knowing the activity that the athlete was engaged in will help. For example, was the athlete coming down from a rebound in basketball; did he or she catch a cross-country ski tip while going downhill? In chronic instability there frequently is very little provocation to injury and very little pain. Essentially, the ligaments are incompetent, and any torsional stress to the ankle will result in subluxation or dislocation.

The amount of swelling present relative to the time of injury is important. Minimal swelling immediately after an injury is not as important a barometer of the extent of injury compared with the amount of swelling after 24 hours. An isolated first time grade III injury to the ATF can result in swelling that increases during an on-the-field examination. Bleeding and edema from disrupted tissues will cause progressive swelling and pain over 24 hours.

If possible, gently apply finger point pressure to the anatomic structures that may be involved in the sprain and to those areas in which associated injury can occur. It is also helpful to thoroughly examine the opposite ankle first, to obtain a baseline of stability. Then apply simple finger pressure in the region of the deltoid ligament, the ATF, the CFL, the PTF, the fibula, the peroneal sheath, the fifth metatarsal, the medial malleolus, and the syndesmosis region. If syndesmosis tenderness is present, palpate the fibula proximally looking for a Maisonneuve fracture. This gentle but specific anatomic examination will give clues as to what is injured and what is not. It will also gain the patient's confidence and allow performance of one stress test in situations where there is not a lot of swelling and spasm.

The anterior drawer test should be performed with the patient sitting, the knee bent, and the ankle plantarflexed in a position of comfort. Flexing the knee relaxes the posterior gastrocnemius. Plantarflexing the ankle relaxes the peroneal tendons. The tibia is braced with one hand while the hindfoot is gently pulled forward (Fig. 1). The amount of anterior translation is compared to that on the opposite side. Next, the hindfoot is grasped, still with the opposite hand holding the lower leg. Gently invert the hindfoot.

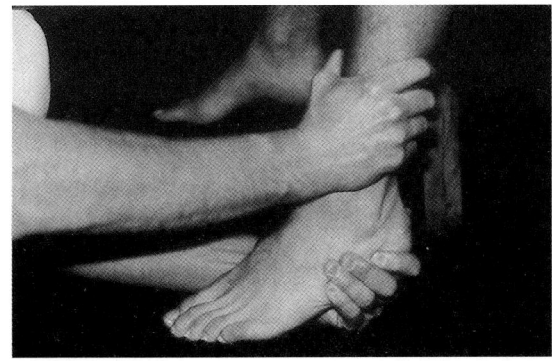

**FIGURE 1**
An illustration of a gentle anterior drawer test with the knee flexed and the ankle plantarflexed.

If a great deal of swelling and spasm are present, these tests should not be performed. The degree of joint effusion and swelling should be regarded as prima fascia evidence that ligament rupture has occurred. Treatment should be based on this assumption; further painful stress testing, arthrography, or stress testing under anesthesia is not necessary.

Radiographic studies for a grade II or III injury should start with an anteroposterior (AP) and a lateral radiograph. If there is no focal bone tenderness, grade I sprains generally do not require a radiograph of the ankle. The routine use of computed tomography (CT), magnetic resonance imaging (MRI), or technetium 99 bone scanning is not warranted in evaluation of a patient's acute ankle sprain. These studies are of value only when associated pathology is suspected. A mortise view in maximum dorsiflexion and plantarflexion may reveal talar dome lesions. The mortise and oblique views can be considered in more severe injuries, but for routine sprains, the AP and lateral views usually are adequate.

Stress testing, even under anesthesia, does not have a great deal of reliability.[1] Similarly, the routine use of arthrography or comparison Telos device stress testing often yields inconclusive results. This is particularly true in an acute sprain in which pain and spasm prevent relaxation. Treatment considerations should be based on the clinical presentation, the degree of hemorrhage and swelling, as well as a history of chronic sprains. Treatment should be based on the extent of the sprain and whether or not associated pathology is present. For example, the AP and lateral radiographs are appropriate for routine screening, additional views or CT would be appropriate for more severe or chronic injuries.

## TREATMENT

### Nonsurgical Treatment

Nonsurgical treatment of an acute ankle sprain is preferred unless associated pathology is present. Dislocations, fractures, or peroneal tendon tears will be a factor in this decision process. In the absence of associated pathology or a history of chronic sprains, nonsurgical treatment has been shown to be the safest and most efficacious. Treatment includes reduction of pain and swelling, adequate immobilization to allow ligament fibers to reappose and heal, and rehabilitation of the peroneal muscles with restoration of normal ankle motion.

Grade I sprains generally will not require professional treatment or rehabilitation. The ankle remains stable and associated injury is rare. Use of ice, elevation, over-the-counter anti-inflammatory medication, and weightbearing depend on patient judgment and symptoms of pain. The resumption of sports may occur with a prophylactic ankle brace or supportive tape. A good test for return to sports is when a patient can single-leg hop on the involved ankle without difficulty.

**Phase I Treatment and Rehabilitation** Grade II and III ankle sprains are treated similarly, although short-term immobilization may be helpful. I prefer to use standard early treatment modalities following the acronym of RICE (rest, ice, compression, and elevation). This format allows for early management of bleeding and edema, the reduction of which is imperative in treatment. I prefer initial immobilization in a boot walker until the swelling subsides, although an ankle brace may also be used. The boot walker may be removed to allow for an ice compress or ice massage for 20 minutes, four times a day during the 48-hour swelling phase of the patient's injury. Elastic compression or pneumatic compression devices can be added during the course of this early treatment. Although crutches may be necessary initially as a result of pain, the boot walker or ankle brace will protect the injured ligaments and allow for earlier weightbearing. Reduction of swelling and protective immobilization of the ankle are the goals of treatment. Once the pain, edema, and old blood have subsided, early motion can be initiated.

**Phase II Treatment and Rehabilitation** When swelling has subsided, typically between 1 and 3 weeks, the ankle still requires ligament protection by boot walker or brace. However, it is now time to begin the active component of rehabilitation that will restore proprioception, peroneal muscle strength, and joint motion. Voluntary active and gentle passive ankle motion should be initiated. Using the toes to curl a small towel on the floor assists in regaining extensor and flexor tendon function. The proprioception board with graduated ball sizes has been shown to offer great benefit in proprioceptive and strengthening rehabilitation (Fig. 2). Isometric and isotonic eversion resistance exercises strengthen the peroneal muscles. This process may take between 4 and 10 weeks before the patient is ready to move to phase III.

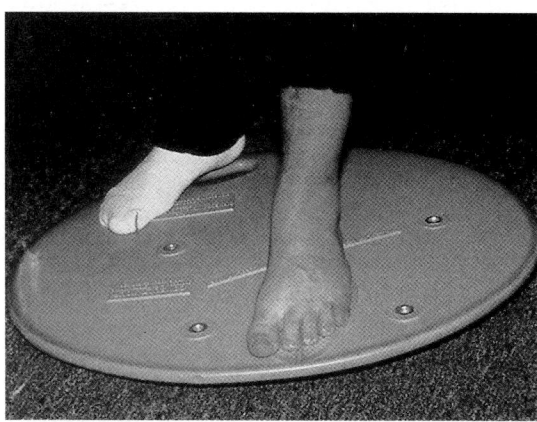

**FIGURE 2**
The proprioception board with variable-sized balls used for proprioceptive and strengthening rehabilitation. The patient stands on the affected ankle, rolling the board around in a circle.

**Phase III Treatment and Rehabilitation** Between 3 and 6 weeks, the patient's ankle stability should be the same as that of the opposite side. It is now time to begin sports-specific rehabilitation. A protective functional brace or trainer-applied taping before exercise is important. The brace or tape offers greater stability and the skin contact increases proprioceptive awareness. Activity should be graduated. Walking graduates to brisk walking; brisk walking graduates to walking on an incline. This activity is then graduated to jogging. Eversion exercises using exercise-resistance machines, surgical tubing or "Sport Cord," or repetitive eversion of the ankle while hanging it over the end of a sofa or table should be continued. These exercises can be enhanced by the therapist's use of a slide board for lateral sliding and by the use of a small trampoline. When the patient can easily and independently perform single-leg hopping, rehabilitation is complete.

Patients who fail to progress with rehabilitation or who have persistent symptoms 3 months after initial injury may have additional associated pathology.

# ANATOMIC VARIATIONS PREDISPOSING TO ANKLE SPRAINS

## STRUCTURAL ANATOMY

There are specific anatomic variations of the ankle mortise that can predispose an athlete to repeated sprains. The normal ankle mortise is saddle-shaped. The medial and lateral malleoli are generally opposite each other, with the dome-shaped talus secure in the concave-shaped tibial plafond. Medial, lateral, or posterior translation is opposed by the respective malleoli. The fibula is dynamic during gait; it is pulled distally through eccentric lengthening approximately 2.5 mm by the contracting flexors and peroneal muscles that stabilize the foot during the stance phase[2] (Fig. 3). The lateral mortise becomes deeper during the period of maximum stance phase stress, and during the dorsiflexion period of the stance phase, the wider portion of the talus rotates into the mortise and the fibula translates laterally, approx-

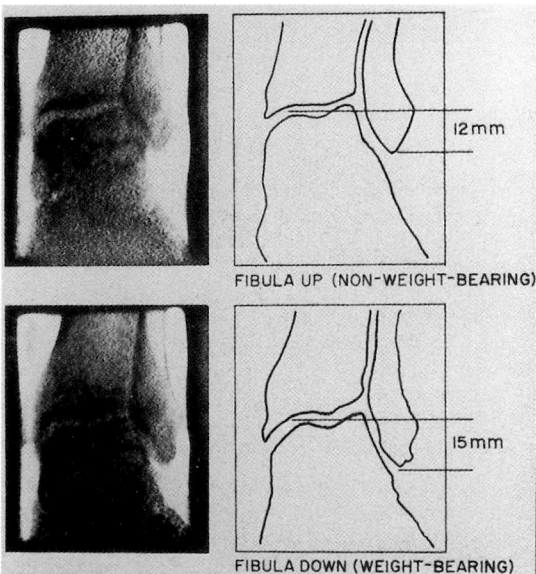

**FIGURE 3**
A diagrammatic illustration of the dynamic nature of fibular motion associated with contraindication of the posterior flexors of the foot. (Reproduced with permission from Weinert CR Jr, McMaster JH, Scranton PE Jr, Ferguson RJ: *Foot Science: Human Fibular Dynamics.* Philadelphia, PA, WB Saunders, pp 106.)

imately 1.5 mm, to accommodate the wider anterior talar dome. Variations in the anatomic structures or dynamic muscular control or failure of the ligament to heal, will predispose to reinjury.

## PERONEAL MUSCLES

The peroneal muscles are the primary dynamic muscular stabilizers of the ankle. Their role in rehabilitation has been well described. However, certain patients demonstrate deficient proprioception and peroneal muscular deficiency, and this possibility must be evaluated in patients with recurrent sprains.[3,4] Electromyography and nerve conduction tests are a reasonable means of evaluating this possibility. Patients with progressive neurologic disorders, such as Charcot-Marie-Tooth disease, have poor peroneal muscle function, especially peroneus brevis, and a predisposition to recurrent ankle sprains. This predisposition exists because hindfoot varus combines with the weakened peroneals to increase the likelihood of an inversion

injury. Patients with peroneal nerve injuries also will be vulnerable. Finally, the muscle itself may be weakened by interstitial tears or tears of the tendon at the time of injury, which will then predispose to reinjury.

## VARUS TIBIAL PLAFOND OR HINDFOOT

Patients with a varus tibial plafond or varus hindfoot have an increased likelihood of recurrent sprains (Fig. 4). Sugimoto and associates[5] described this congenital variation of a varus plafond, noting that because the hindfeet of these patients were not in valgus, the vector of forces was more medial and likely to cause an inversion sprain. It has also been noted that the cavus foot, with a depressed first ray and varus heel, is structurally prone to lateral ankle sprains.[6] Clearly, when the vector of forces is centered medial to the center of the mortise, the lateral ankle is vulnerable.

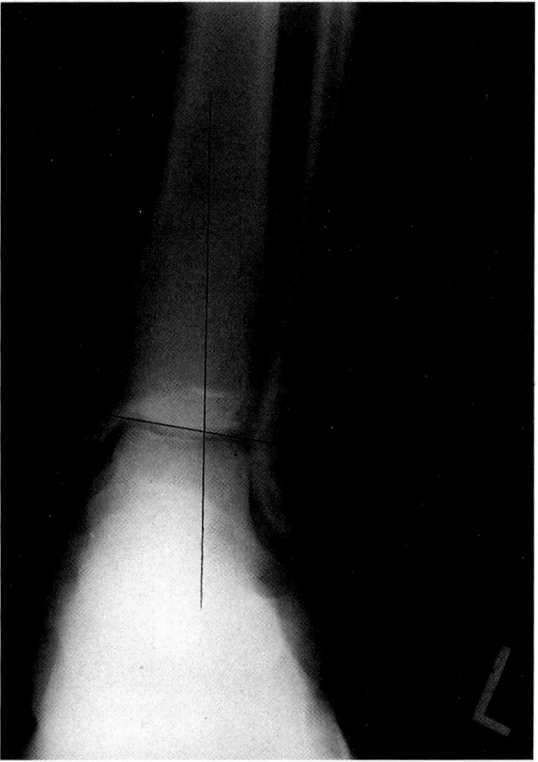

**FIGURE 4**
A standing anteroposterior radiograph of an ankle with a varus heel in a patient with chronic ankle instability.

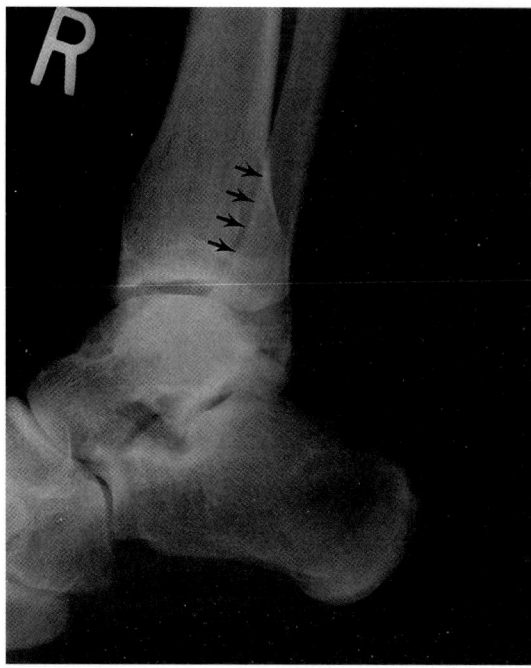

**FIGURE 5**
A lateral radiograph of a patient's chronically sprained ankle in which the fibula is more posteriorly positioned. The mortise is more "opened," leading to greater vulnerability to a sprain.

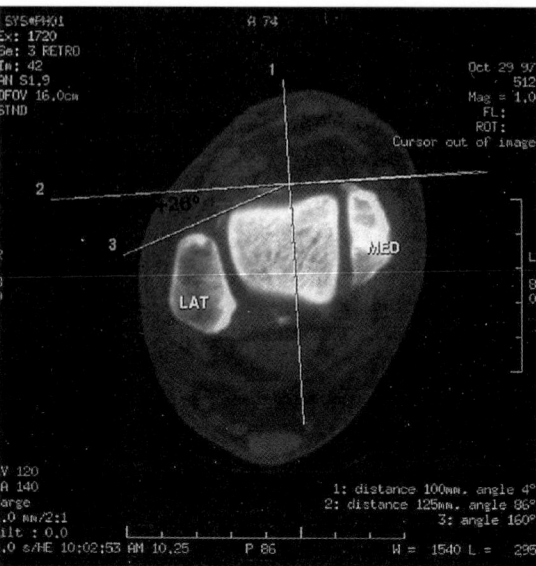

**FIGURE 6**
A computed tomogram illustrating a posteriorly positioned fibula.

## POSTERIORLY POSITIONED FIBULA

The final variation is the posteriorly positioned fibula. When the malleoli are directly opposite each other, the saddle-like mortise has maximum structural stability. However, there is a 38° range of variation in the posterior position of the fibula relative to the medial malleolus[7] (Fig. 5). In some patients, the fibula is positioned anterior to the medial malleolus, while in others it is positioned posteriorly up to 26° (Fig. 6). This posterior positioning "opens" the mortise, making it structurally more vulnerable to recurrent sprains of the lateral ankle ligament complex. These predisposing variations to ankle reinjury are summarized in Outline 1.

## ANKLE INSTABILITY

Patients with chronic ankle instability, if untreated, will often go on to develop arthritic degeneration. It is important to evaluate clinically unstable patients for the previously mentioned

**OUTLINE 1**

**ANATOMIC AND FUNCTIONAL FACTORS ASSOCIATED WITH ANKLE SPRAINS**

1. Proprioceptive deficiency
2. Peroneal muscular weakness
3. Peroneal tendon tears
4. Varus tibial plafond
5. Varus hindfoot
6. Posteriorly positioned fibula

predisposing factors before considering surgery. For example, an ankle ligament stabilization procedure performed in the presence of severe hindfoot varus will most likely fail. The varus calcaneus must be corrected by a Dwyer or laterally displacing calcaneal osteotomy. The presence of loose bodies or degenerative spurs is not a contradiction to a stabilization procedure. The loose bodies and spurs should be debrided at the time of surgery (Fig. 7). It is important not to create more articular damage than already exists. Tibial or talar spurs should be removed carefully with beveled instruments so as not to further damage

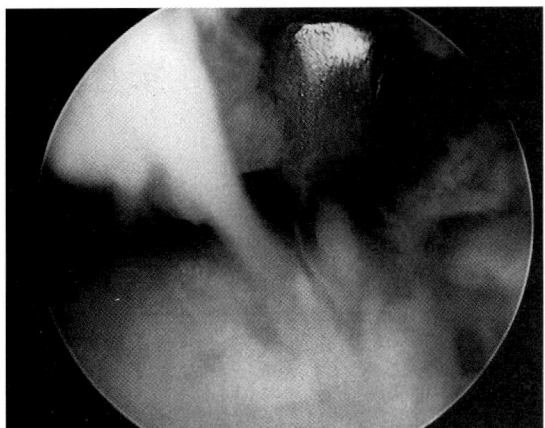

**FIGURE 7**
A small joint osteotome with beveled edges is used for tibial spur debridement. The bevel protects the talar articular surface.

articular surfaces. These spurs limit dorsiflexion and impair ankle function and patient recovery. The presence of a varus plafond or posteriorly positioned fibula does not require osseous correction. However, additional brace protection and prolonged peroneal rehabilitation may be required to secure an effective repair.

## SURGICAL TREATMENT

Patients with a primary grade III ankle sprain and an avulsed fragment of bone from the joint that would impair recovery should undergo primary repair. Patients with a history of repetitive sprains and clinically obvious instability also require stabilization. The following procedures for treating chronic instability have been successful in my experience.

### BRÖSTROM PROCEDURE

Hamilton and associates described the Gould modification of the Bröstrom procedure.[8-10] This procedure incorporates the extensor retinaculum into the repair of the imbricated ankle ligament(s), restoring anatomic stability while perhaps tightening to some degree the subtalar joint. It has the advantage of being a simple anatomic repair, it is performed on an outpatient basis, and rehabilitation is similar to phases II and III for an acute sprain.

The operation is performed with the anesthetized patient either lying on his or her contralateral side on a vacuum "bean bag" or with a large bolster under the ipsilateral hip. This position allows the ankle to be rolled over for easy lateral observation. Anesthesia is either by general or spinal anesthetic.

The procedure is carried out as follows: Inspect the ankle and the superficial anatomic landmarks. Pull the foot into adduction by grasping the lateral toes. As this is done, look for the course of the superficial peroneal nerve and its branches so that they can be avoided. Perform anterior drawer and varus stress testing on both limbs to gauge the required tightness of repair. The incision should be longitudinal, allowing access to the anterior ankle joint, the ATF, and the CFL while avoiding the superficial peroneal nerves (Fig. 8). Identify and mobilize the extensor retinaculum (Fig. 9). Transect the remnants of the anterior talofibular ligament at its midpoint. In patients with chronic instability, this usually represents an amorphous mass of fibrous scar tissue and may be quite attenuated. Explore the ankle and remove spurs or loose bodies.[11] Perform varus stress testing under direct vision. If the CFL is incompetent, identify the stretched ligament and divide it. Use a 0 or #1 absorbable suture to imbricate these ligaments in a "vest-over-pants" fashion (Fig. 10). Incorporate the superior border

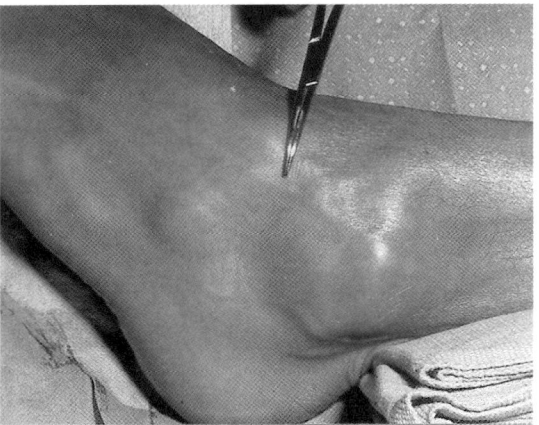

**FIGURE 8**
The hemostat points to the superficial peroneal nerve on a left ankle. The surgical incision should protect this nerve.

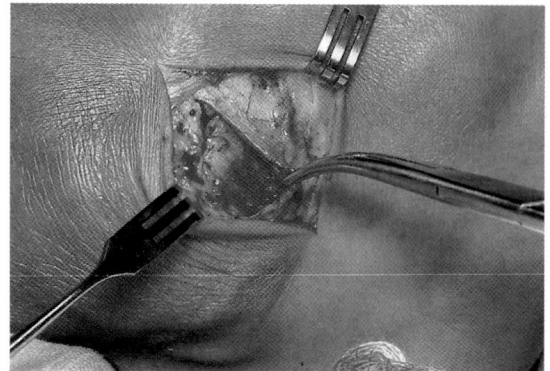

**FIGURE 9**
The extensor retinaculum on a right ankle is identified and protected so it may be incorporated into the reconstruction.

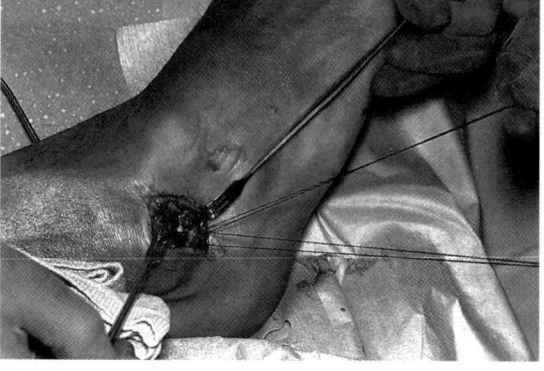

**FIGURE 10**
The "vest-over-pants" imbrication on a right ankle of the cut ends of the anterior talofibular ligament with a 0 suture.

of the extensor retinaculum into this reconstruction. Nonabsorbable sutures can cause painful snapping and synovitis as they rub over the corner of the lateral talus. Make sure to avoid the superficial peroneal nerve and its branches during closure. The patient's wound is infiltrated with 0.25% bipuvicaine hydrochloride with epinephrine and the patient is then discharged in a boot walker with crutches.

The wound should be examined 10 to 14 days postoperatively. If there are no problems with healing, the wound is redressed, the boot walker reapplied, and graduated weightbearing initiated. At 3 weeks postoperatively, the patient is reexamined. If the reconstruction resists gentle varus and anterior stressing, the boot walker is discontinued. A brace is applied and phase II followed by phase III rehabilitation is begun.

## ALTERNATIVE SURGICAL PROCEDURES

Variations in ligament pathology will dictate the need for some degree of flexibility in the surgical approach. For example, the ATF or CFL may have avulsed off its origin at the fibula. The ligament itself is competent and intact; only the origin is incompetent. In this case, the bone fragment should be excised, and the fibular origin bone should be freshened with a small osteotome. Two suture anchors should be drilled into this region, taking care not to penetrate the talofibular joint. With the anchors secure, the suture portion is used to reattach the respective ligament. The extensor retinaculum may be incorporated into this repair, particularly if other anatomic predisposing factors such as a varus tibial plafond or posterior fibula are present. This suture anchor reconstruction approach also may be used on the talus if the distal ATFL insertion has been avulsed.

On rare occasions, when there is inadequate ligament available for a Bröstrom-type reconstruction, a so-called "weaving procedure" is indicated. A variety of these procedures have been described, many of which have been demonstrated to be efficacious.[12] In my opinion, the Chrisman-Snook procedure[13] has been most satisfactory.

## CHRISMAN-SNOOK PROCEDURE

The patient is anesthetized with either spinal or general anesthesia, and is placed either on a "bean bag" under the contralateral hip or supine with an adequate ipsilateral bolster to roll the involved ankle over for easy exposure. The initial longitudinal incision is similar to that for the Bröstrom procedure. When the absence of suitable reconstructive tissue is confirmed, the incision is expanded proximally to expose the lateral fibula and peroneal tendons, and distally to expose the lateral calcaneus and subtalar joint. After identifying the peroneus brevis tendon, inspect it, looking for longitudinal tears. If a tear is present, develop it further so that half the per-

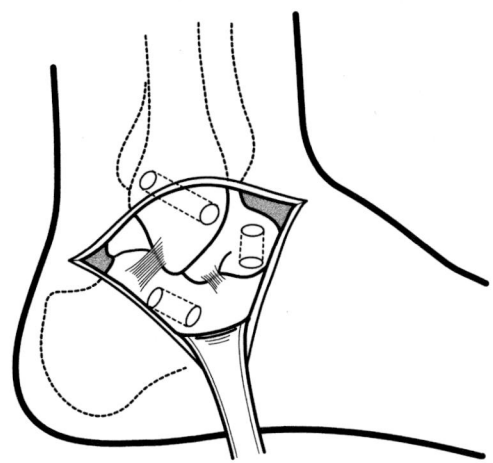

**FIGURE 11**
The diagrammatic illustration of the method of drilling the fibular, talar, and calcaneal holes for the passage of half the peroneus brevis tendon from top through the fibula, then through the talus, and finally through the calcaneus. The skin incision is longitudinal-oblique, not the diagrammatic exposure shown here.

oneus brevis is split off from its insertion on the base of the fifth metatarsal, running up to the proximal musculotendinosis junction. Protect the sural nerve. Determine the areas on the talus and calcaneus where the incompetent ligaments used to attach. Using a small drill and power burrs, drill obliquely through the fibula from posterior to anterior, exiting anteriorly at the origin of the ATF. Then drill a hole at the talus insertion point, which is distal to the talofibular joint, and out the bottom of the talus. Finally, drill two holes 1 cm apart into the calcaneus (Fig. 11). With a "whip stitch" of 0 suture around the tip of the tendon strip, pull the strip from the fibula through the talus and then through the calcaneus, attaching it to the fibula. Suture anchors can help.

Make sure the reconstruction is secure, but not so tight as to have locked the subtalar joint. The surgeon should make sure that subtalar movement is not restricted, while at the same time the anterior and varus stress testing of the ankle is secure. A drain may be required. A compression dressing and boot walker are applied. There usually is too much pain for this operation to be performed on an outpatient basis. The dressing may be changed and the drain pulled at discharge. The patient is kept nonweightbearing for 3 weeks and then weightbearing in the boot walker for another 3 weeks. Phase II rehabilitation begins at the fourth week after surgery.

## SYNDESMOSIS INJURIES

Injuries to the ligaments that form the ankle syndesmosis are often referred to as a "high ankle sprain." Such an injury may occur with or without a concomitant ankle sprain. If this diagnosis is missed, the injury will result in months of pain and inability to perform athletically.

The anatomy of the syndesmosis ligaments is illustrated in Figure 12.[14] The anterior tibiofibular ligament, syndesmosis, and posterior tibiofibular ligament make up the complex that provides mortise stability, yet allows the up and down and lateral fibular translatory motions of normal gait. In addition, the interosseous membrane runs between the entire length of the fibula and tibia, providing additional load transference and stability (Fig. 13).

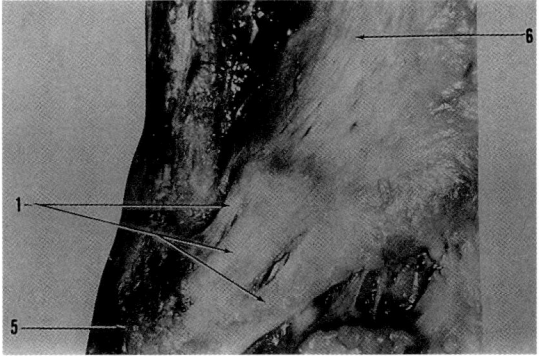

**FIGURE 12**
The thick posterior tibiofibular syndesmosis ligament (1). Note the separate bundles that insert on the fibula anteriorly (5); an inferior bundle can sometimes painfully abrade the lateral dome of the talus (Bassett's lesion). (Reproduced with permission from Sarrafian SK: *Anatomy of the Foot and Ankle: Descriptive, Topographic, Functional.* Philadelphia, PA, JB Lippincott, 1983, pp 143–198.)

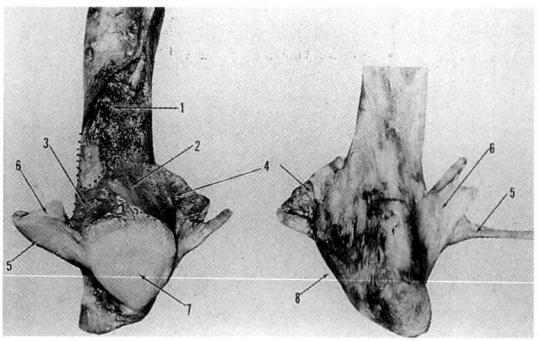

**FIGURE 13**
The medial and lateral view of the distal fibula dissection with anterior tibiofibular (5,6), posterior tibiofibular (4), and interosseous ligaments (1). (Reproduced with permission from Sarrafian SK: *Anatomy of the Foot and Ankle: Descriptive, Topographic, Functional.* Philadelphia, PA, JB Lippincott, 1983, pp 35–106.)

## MECHANISMS OF INJURY

The mechanisms of injury are forced dorsiflexion of the ankle, external rotation of the leg, or abduction of the foot. These injuries generally occur only in association with either pivoting and cutting sports or trauma. For example, an athlete may have a foot planted on the ground as someone falls on the athlete from behind. The ankle is forced into extreme dorsiflexion, and the wide, anterior portion of the talus forces a partial tear of the anterior fibers of the anterior tibiofibular ligament. With external rotation injuries, the athlete's foot is fixed to the turf at the instant the athlete pivots or cuts toward the opposite side. The external rotation torque can progressively tear the anterior tibiofibular ligament, the syndesmosis, and the posterior tibiofibular ligament. If the interosseous membrane is torn from inferior to superior, as the tear extends proximally and the anterior perforating peroneal artery is disrupted, a compartment syndrome can occur. As the tear advances up the interosseous ligament, the forces may cause the proximal fibula to turn outward, creating a Maisonneuve fracture (Fig. 14). Pure abduction forces that disrupt only the syndesmosis complex are rare but can occur. Usually, disruption of the medial deltoid ligament or medial malleolar avulsion fracture occurs at the same time as disruption and spread of the entire syndesmosis.

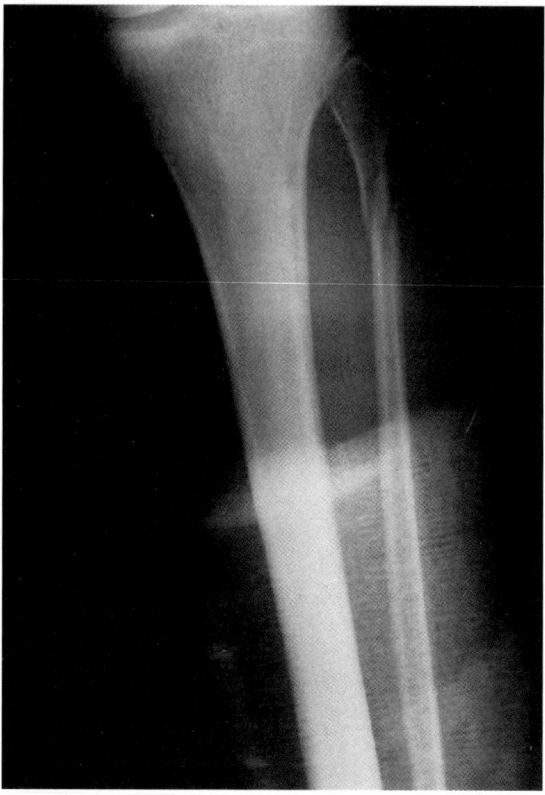

**FIGURE 14**
An anteroposterior radiograph of the proximal fibula in a patient who was diagnosed with a severe ankle sprain. As the tear advances up the interosseous ligment, Maisonneuve fracture occurs. This type of fracture represents the exit point of the forces that tore the entire interosseous membrane before spiraling out the proximal fibula.

## PHYSICAL FINDINGS AND RADIOGRAPHIC EVALUATION

The single most reliable physical findings are swelling and discrete point tenderness over the anterior tibiofibular ligament. Direct finger pressure will confirm these findings (Fig. 15). Compressing the fibula against the tibia can produce pain as these torn ligaments are stressed, and this represents a positive "squeeze" test (Fig. 16). If the foot is gently externally rotated while the lower leg is held stationary, exquisite pain at the syndesmosis will again confirm injury (Fig. 17). Painful dorsiflexion should arouse suspicion as well as pain medially at the deltoid ligament. If the proximal fibula is painful, a radiograph may con-

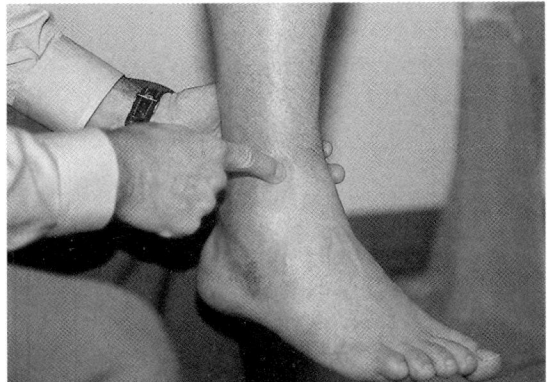

**FIGURE 15**
Direct pressure over the anterior syndesmosis region.

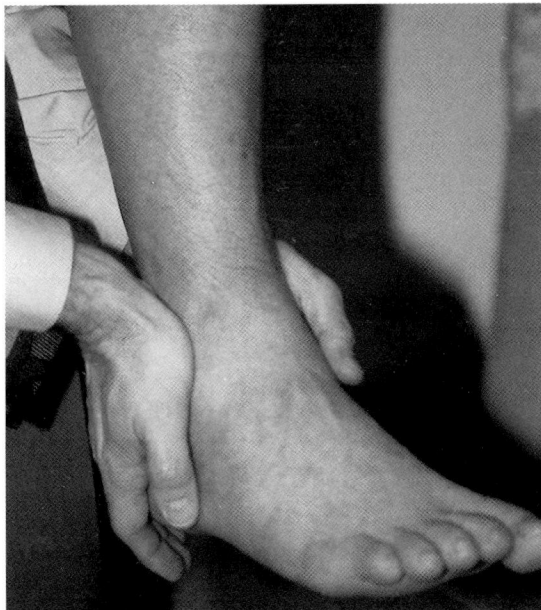

**FIGURE 16**
Direct compression of the distal fibula against the tibia can produce pain. In the absence of radiographic evidence of fracture, this is strongly suggestive of syndesmosis injury.

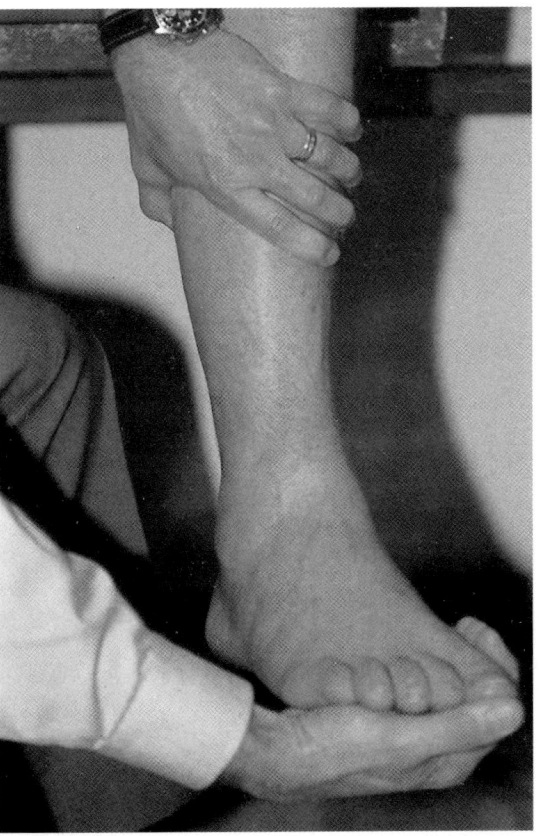

**FIGURE 17**
The external rotation stress test. Severe anterior syndesmosis pain confirms the syndesmosis injury.

firm complete syndesmosis disruption with a concomitant Maisonneuve fracture. In this instance, the fibula may have "hinged posteriorly," the anterior tibiofibular and interosseous ligaments ruptured, with the resulting forces spiraling out the proximal fibula. Note that the posterior tibiofibular ligament may still be intact.

Plain AP and lateral radiographs may be deceiving. If the extent of injury seen on the radiographs does not seem appropriate, additional studies should be done. An external rotation and abduction stress test done while the patient is under anesthesia will confirm syndesmosis instability (Fig. 18). Axial views on a MRI are also valuable. The T2-weighted images will show the extent of ligament disruption (Fig. 19). A CT scan with bilateral transverse views through the syndesmosis can be helpful in detecting subtle widening between the fibula and tibia. An isolated CT scan will not show any comparison relationships, whereas bilateral scans can be helpful in assessing damage and predicting a return to athletics or work.

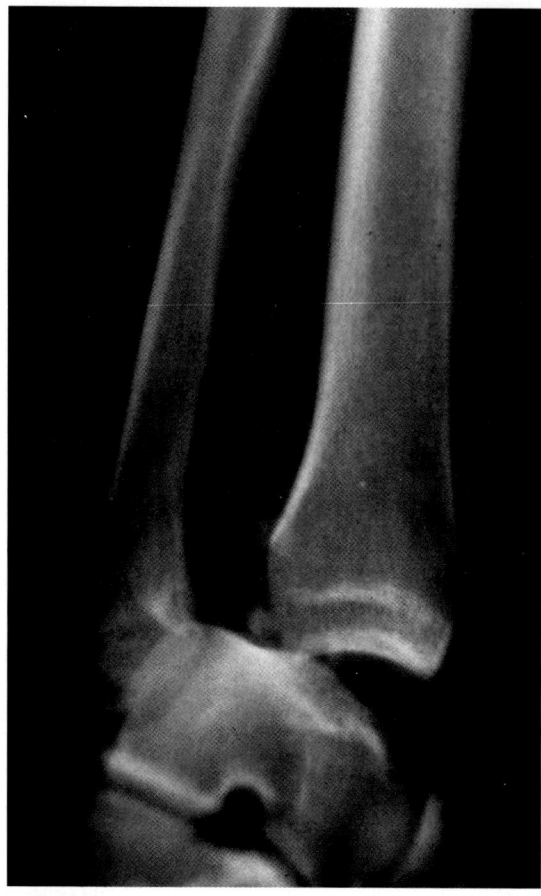

**FIGURE 18**
An external rotation stress test radiograph taken with the patient under anesthesia. (Photo courtesy of Carol C. Teitz MD, Seattle, WA.)

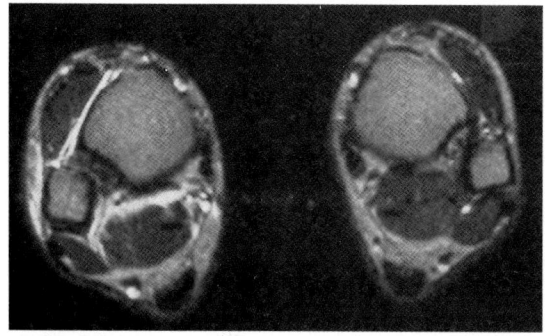

**FIGURE 19**
An axial T2-weighted magnetic resonance image of a football player who has had a grade II/III anterior syndesmosis injury on the right ankle. Note the increased signal in the anterior compartment.

## CLASSIFICATION

As in ankle sprains, syndesmosis injuries have been classified into grades I, II, and III. Again, this descriptive classification is relevant only to the ligamentous component of the injury. Adjacent periarticular injuries should be investigated by physical examination and appropriate imaging studies. A grade I injury occurs with either forced dorsiflexion or external rotation. Swelling is minimal or absent. There is point tenderness anteriorly only at the anterior tibiofibular ligament. Ambulation is not difficult. No treatment is necessary unless competitive athletic activity is desired. Protective taping with a ¼" heel lift and an external shoe "spat" may provide protection and the ability to return to sport.

The grade II injury is unstable. The entire anterior tibiofibular ligament has been torn along with the inferior interosseous ligament. The posterior tibiofibular ligament is intact. Swelling and significant pain are apparent. The patient can point to the area of pain (point test), and results of squeeze and external rotational stress tests are positive. Ambulation is difficult. Dorsiflexion of the ankle is painful.

The grade III injury represents a serious injury that demands an accurate diagnosis, compartment monitoring, and surgical fixation. Significant swelling is present. The radiographs may be deceiving. The clear space may match the opposite side, but a lateral external rotational stress radiograph under anesthesia will show obvious posterior fibular migration. A transfibular syndesmosis screw will be necessary; it is applied either under direct vision or percutaneously with a cannulated screw (Fig. 20). If the reduction is inadequate, it is possible that the deltoid ligament may be avulsed and flipped into the medial ankle. This blocks reduction. This situation must be corrected by a medial arthrotomy and direct repair.

## TREATMENT

The management of grade I, II, and III injuries depends on an accurate diagnosis. Once the physical and radiologic assessments are complete a treatment plan can be established.

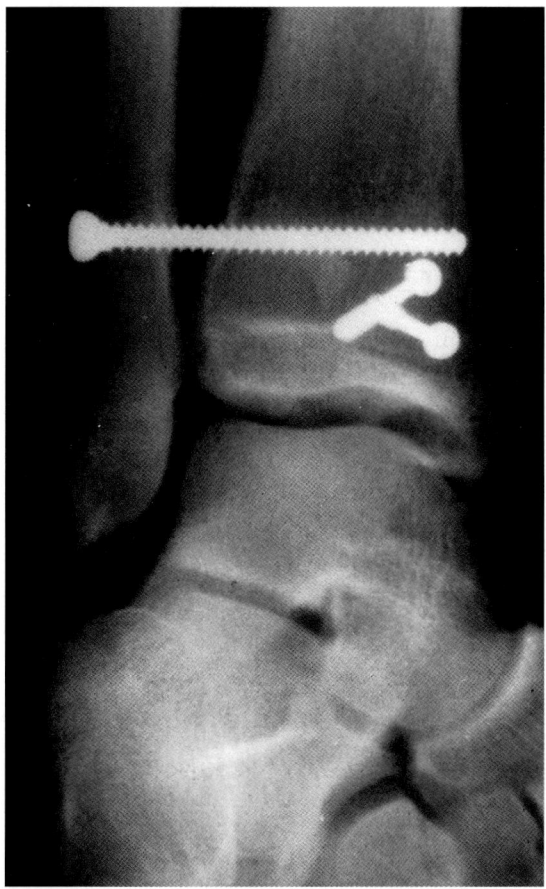

**FIGURE 20**
A postreduction radiograph of the patient seen in Figure 18. Medial small fragment screws secure avulsed medial bone fragments and the attached deltoid ligament. (Photo courtesy of Carol C. Teitz MD, Seattle, WA.)

Patient education is most important. The patient and, if necessary, coaches need to understand that the syndesmosis injury is not a simple sprained ankle. In a competitive athlete, a grade II or III injury will probably mean loss of the season. A grade I injury will probably result in a 3- to 6-week absence from sports.

A grade I injury may require nonweightbearing for 10 days to 3 weeks, depending on pain and symptoms. Phase II and III rehabilitation then follows with "clamshell" taping using horseshoe moleskin applied in a stirrup fashion and overtaped with a conventional basketweave technique or bracing to support the anterior syndesmosis. A 1-cm, felt heel lift will assist in preventing the wider anterior talus from irritating the anterior mortise during rehabilitation.

Grade II syndesmosis injuries require nonweightbearing for at least 3 weeks and up to 6 weeks. Again, progressive phase II and III rehabilitation is initiated. The boot walker is worn for at least 6 weeks, followed by a clamshell brace.

Grade III syndesmosis injuries require stabilization. A transfibular 3 cortex cannulated 6.5-mm or 7.3-mm cancellous screw placed 1 cm above the ankle joint should be used to effect reduction. The screw should be tightened down with the ankle in dorsiflexion to prevent the talus from impinging in the ankle mortise during the extreme of dorsiflexion. The patient should be nonweightbearing for 6 weeks, but ankle motion out of the brace is allowed after 3 weeks. Weightbearing can commence in the boot walker for the second 6 weeks; after 12 weeks the syndesmosis screw can be removed on an outpatient basis. Phase II and III rehabilitation then is begun.

One rare complication of syndesmosis injuries is interosseous ligament ossification (Fig. 21). It is rarely seen, and tibiofibular motion generally is not restricted, even if heterotopic bone forms. If a tibiofibular synostosis forms, normal fibular motion at the ankle joint is restricted. Anterior ankle pain commonly is associated with the mortise restriction, because the wider anterior talus cannot fit in the mortise during dorsiflexion.[15] Symptomatic tibiofibular synostoses require resection, packing in bone wax over the cut tibial and fibular surfaces, and an interposed fat graft to prevent recurrence.

## CHRONIC DIASTASIS

Chronic syndesmosis instability is rarely encountered. Medial deltoid ligament laxity must be a concomitant finding. Thus repair is directed toward both medial stabilization and lateral soft-tissue reconstruction. Because the deltoid ligament has both deep and superficial insertional points on the talus and calcaneus, the ligament should be repaired more proximally. The ligament may be exposed using a longitudinal incision, centered over the medial malleolus.

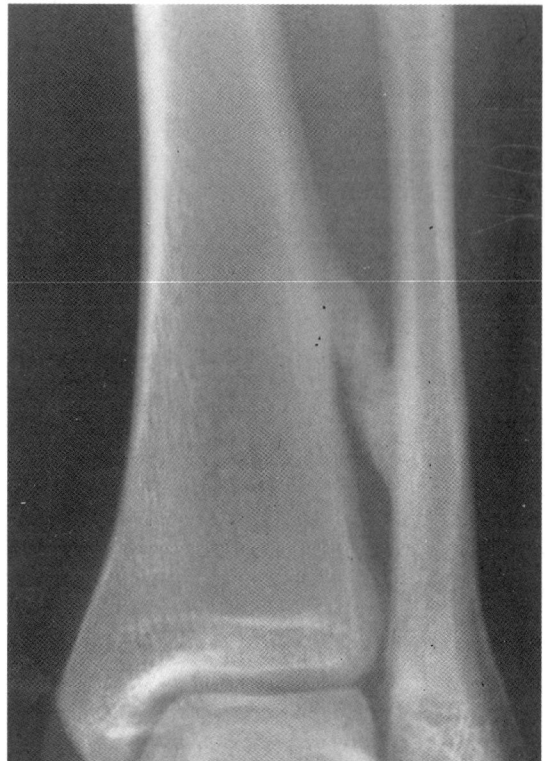

**FIGURE 21**
A painful complete tibiofibular synostosis that has formed in a patient after a "high ankle sprain." (Reproduced with permission from McMaster JH, Scranton PE: Tibiofibular synostosis: A cause of ankle disability. *Clin Orthop* 1975;111:172–174.)

laxity. This section also may be imbricated using a "vest-over-pants" suture. Nonabsorbable sutures, either 0 or #1, should be used. Closure is routine. The foot is immobilized in a boot walker, no weightbearing is allowed for 6 weeks, then weightbearing is allowed for 6 more weeks. The transfibular screw is removed, and phase II and III rehabilitation is begun.

The importance and gravity of syndesmosis injuries is shown in Figure 22. Chronic syndesmosis instability in combination with the repetitive shear forces on the talocrural joint can lead to complete arthrosis of the joint, requiring arthrodesis.

## PERONEAL TENDON INJURIES

A substantial spectrum of pathology can occur in association with the peroneal tendons (Outline 2).

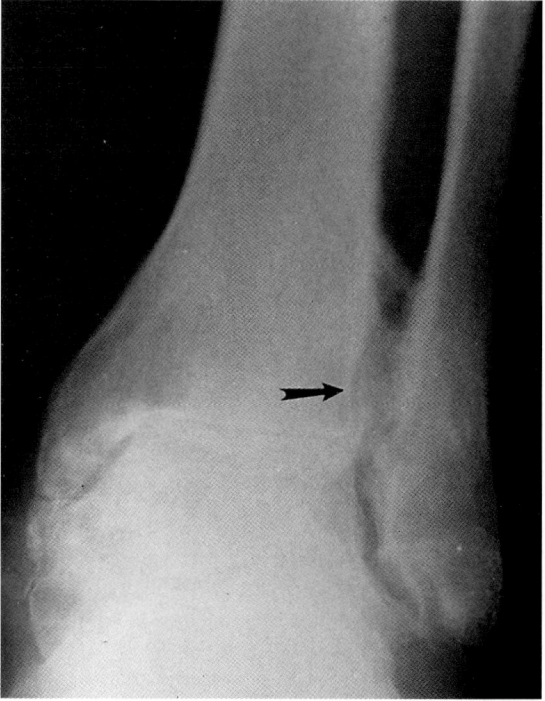

**FIGURE 22**
An anteroposterior radiograph of the ankle of a patient 8 years after severe syndesmosis disruption. Note the talocrural arthrosis and interosseous ossification.

When the anterior and posterior deltoid borders have been defined, inspect the medial anterior joint, removing fibrous tissue if encountered. Then direct attention to the fibular side. A section of peroneus brevis tendon is harvested from distal to proximal and passed through transfibular and tibial drill holes at the level of the anterior syndesmosis. The fibula is transfixed with a transfibular screw. The ankle is dorsiflexed, and the transfibular screw is tightened. The tendon will become a new syndesmosis ligament. It is then passed through the drill holes, pulled out medially, and sutured or stapled on the medial tibia.

Attention is now returned to the deltoid ligament. Its laxity should now be apparent. A transverse section is removed across the width of the

**OUTLINE 2**

**PERONEAL TENDON PATHOLOGY**

1. Peroneal tendon dislocation
2. Peroneal tendon subluxation
3. Peroneus longus or brevis rupture
4. Peroneal tendon longitudinal tear(s)
5. Os peroneum fractures
6. Peroneal tendinitis
7. Peroneal aberrant muscle slip tears
8. Fifth metatarsal base avulsion injuries

Injury to the tendons can be acute in association with a traumatic event or attritional.

The mechanism for injury to the peroneal tendons often comes in combination with an ankle sprain. Supination or external rotation-supination injuries to the ankle lead, at the moment of injury, to violent peroneal muscular contraction in an effort to evert and stabilize the ankle. If the force vectors are greater than the anatomic constraints of the fibular groove and peroneal sheath, the tendons dislocate. If the groove and sheath constraints can resist tendon dislocation, proximal or distal tendon rupture or insertional avulsion can occur. A careful history combined with radiographs and a physical examination will help make the diagnosis.

## PHYSICAL FINDINGS

The most reliable signs for peroneal tendon pathology are pain and swelling over the course of the tendons.[16] Crepitance is sometimes palpable in the peroneal sheaths as the patient actively inverts and everts the foot. If longitudinal splits in the tendon(s) are present, pain usually is localized to the fibular groove region because this area is relatively avascular for the tendons, and as they move back and forth around the groove, injury occurs. A snapping sensation can frequently be elicited with active eversion. In addition, with resisted dorsiflexion and eversion, the tendons can be seen to actively dislocate over the corner of the fibula if sheath pathology is present (Fig. 23). This snapping sensation will also produce pain.

The peroneus longus is deep to the peroneus brevis tendon and more protected at the fibula, but it is subject to tears and attritional changes where it crosses inferior to the cuboid bone at the cubital groove (Fig. 24). The os peroneum is sometimes present, and radiographic evidence of os peroneum fragmentation or proximal migration is evidence of peroneus longus ten-

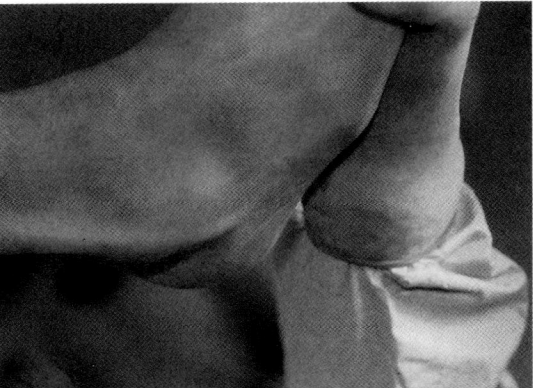

**FIGURE 23**
The peroneal tendons are seen dislocating anteriorly over the fibular border of a right ankle.

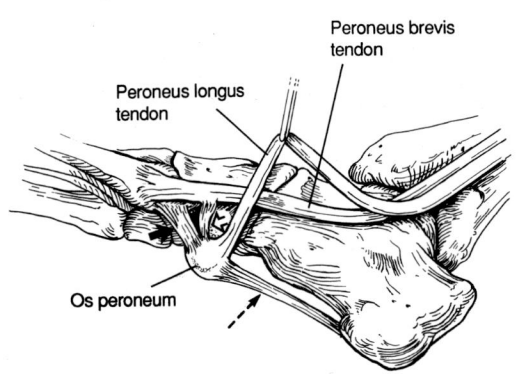

**FIGURE 24**
A diagrammatic illustration of the peroneus brevis tendon and the peroneus longus tendon complete with the enclosed os peroneum. (Reproduced with permission from Sobel M, Mizel MS: Peroneal tendon injury, in Pfeffer GB, Frey CC (eds): *Current Practice in Foot and Ankle Surgery.* New York, NY, McGraw-Hill, 1993, pp 30–56.)

don injury. Significant pain and a mass in the proximal peroneal muscles with weakness on eversion is evidence of a proximal muscle partial or complete tear.

## DIAGNOSTIC MEASURES

As mentioned, weakness to resisted eversion with localized pain and swelling are the most common physical signs associated with peroneal tendon pathology. Radiographs may be helpful, but only if osseous pathology is present. AP and lateral radiographs will reveal the lateral fibular border and the region of the cuboid bone. A fleck of bone avulsed off the lateral fibula will confirm the diagnosis of dislocation of the peroneal tendons. In the lateral plane, fragmentation or proximal migration of the os peroneum will confirm peroneus longus tendon injury. If necessary, a Harris view will reveal the fibular groove and assist in surgical planning if recurrent peroneal tendon dislocation surgery is contemplated.

Peroneal tendon tenography will not reveal meaningful new information that has not been documented during a good history and physical examination. Ultrasonography can confirm tendon injury only. A CT scan is of no benefit in diagnosing these tendon injuries. An MRI scan should not be used routinely; however, it is helpful in ruling out other pathology, such as a ruptured tendon, an aberrant peroneal muscle slip, or chronic tendinitis (Fig. 25).

## TREATMENT OPTIONS

Management of the acute peroneal tendon dislocation can be nonsurgical. If peroneal tendon dislocation is suspected, cast immobilization for 6 weeks is recommended with the ankle held in plantarflexion and inversion for 3 weeks, followed by casting in neutral with no weight bearing for another 3 weeks. Phase II rehabilitation followed by phase III can be initiated at 4 weeks postinjury.

Patients who have 3 months or more of pain, peroneal tendon sheath swelling, snapping sensations, and the feeling that this ankle "gives way" should be managed surgically. Most of the pathology will be localized to the region of the

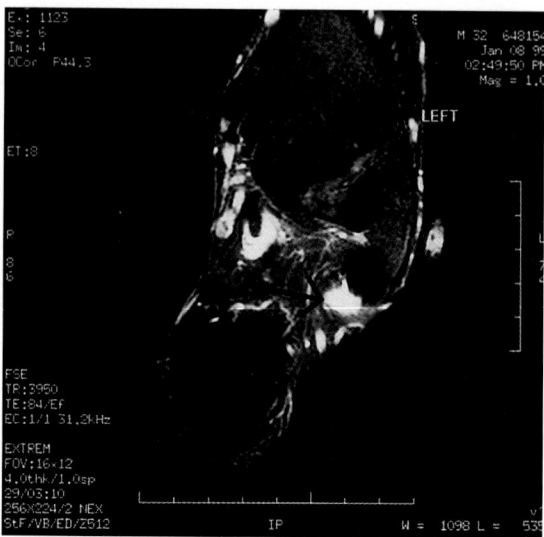

**FIGURE 25**
An axial magnetic resonance image of a patient evaluated for chronic ankle pain after a severe ankle sprain. Note the absent peroneus brevis tendon. (Photo courtesy of John E. McDermott MD, Seattle, WA.)

peroneal groove. A simple exploration performed on an outpatient basis will easily address relevant pathology. Tendon tears, aberrant muscle tears, and subluxations or dislocation can each be treated through the same surgical incision. The surgeon must be ready to deal with one or all three diagnoses at the same operation. The patient's history and clinical examination are the most important determinants in the decision to operate. An MRI may confirm that pathology exists in the fibular groove, but it may overstate or miss concomitant injuries.

## DISLOCATING OR SUBLUXATING PERONEAL TENDONS

Most patients who have this diagnosis have avulsed the sheath anteriorly off the posterior fibular border. A fibrous pseudosheath constrains these tendons after they dislocate anteriorly (Fig. 26). This pseudosheath must be reattached by freshening the posterior border bone and resuturing the sheath with suture anchors (Fig. 27). Immobilization with a boot walker for 3 weeks is followed by phase II and phase III rehabilitation.

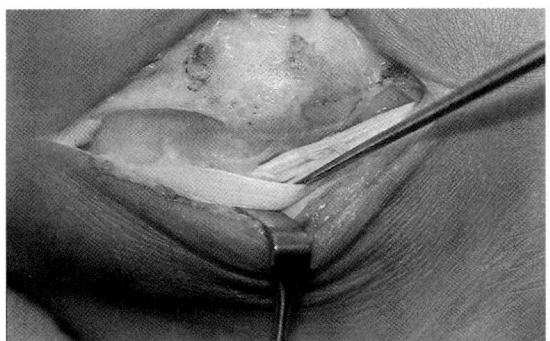

**FIGURE 26**
The fibrous pseudosheath and avulsed peroneal sheath associated with the dislocating peroneal tendons at the corner of the right fibula. Note the torn peroneal tendon.

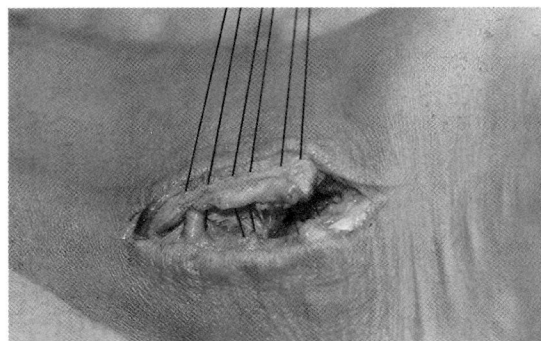

**FIGURE 27**
The use of suture anchors for repair of the sheath to the right fibula.

Groove deepening or reconstruction should be undertaken in the case of an incompetent fibular groove.[17] The sheath may still require reattachment, but if the groove requires deepening, carefully elevate the groove surface with an osteotome and use a power rotary burr to deepen the underlying bone. Then tap back down the groove surface and reattach the sheath. A high percentage of patients with this problem have intra-articular ankle pathology.

Additional techniques in surgical stabilization of dislocating peroneal tendons include either rerouting the tendon under the CFL or trimming down from proximal to distal a flap of Achilles tendon that is attached to the fibula. Both of these techniques are more complex and entail more surgical risks if technical problems occur.

### PERONEAL TENDON TEARS

Symptomatic longitudinal tendon tears of the peroneal tendons are dealt with by repair or resection. A history of chronic symptoms and localized physical findings will indicate if surgical exploration is indicated. Because tomograms generally are not regarded as reliable, both peroneal tendons require complete inspection, plantarflexing and dorsiflexing the ankle to watch them as they move back and forth around the fibular groove. An inferiorly protruding aberrant slip of peroneal muscle with adjacent synovitis will require resection. If only one small longitudinal tendon tear is present, this small tear can be resected. If the tear is midsubstance and substantial or there are multiple tears, a repair is required. I prefer to use a running 4-0 to 2-0 absorbable suture to carry out the repair. Nonabsorbable sutures also have been advocated, but I have seen this cause chronic tenosynovitis. Hence, the resorbable suture is recommended. After 3 weeks of immobilization phase II and phase III rehabilitation are begun.

### DISTAL PERONEUS LONGUS TENDON INJURIES

Localized pain at the cubital groove, with or without a fragmented or migrating os peroneum, is evidence of acute or chronic injury. In my experience most of these present late after months of progressive symptoms. A history of previous ankle sprains or prolonged training in aerobics or running is common. Orthotic management and nonsteroidal anti-inflammatory medications can sometimes be successful. If the tendon is intact but has longitudinal tears or a fragmented os peroneum, the tear should be repaired and the fragmented bone excised. If the peroneus longus tendon is avulsed, it should be tenodesed to the peroneus brevis tendon.

### SUMMARY

The evaluation of soft-tissue ankle injuries requires the assessment of the ligaments and articular and periarticular structures. A patient who has chronic ankle or foot pain after experiencing a major ankle sprain requires evaluation for a variety of diagnoses besides the sprain itself.

## REFERENCES

1. Becker HP, Komischke A, Danz B, Bensel R, Claes L: Stress diagnostics of the sprained ankle: Evaluation of the anterior drawer test with and without anesthesia. *Foot Ankle* 1993;14:459–464.

2. Scranton PE Jr, McMaster JG, Kelly E: Dynamic fibular function: A new concept. *Clin Orthop* 1976;118:76–81.

3. Freeman MA: Treatment of ruptures of the lateral ligament of the ankle. *J Bone Joint Surg* 1965; 47B:661–668.

4. Löfvenberg R, Kärrholm J, Sundelin G, Ahlgren O: Prolonged reaction time in patients with chronic lateral instability of the ankle. *Am J Sports Med* 1995;23:414–417.

5. Sugimoto K, Samoto N, Takakura Y, Tamai S: Varus tilt of the tibial plafond as a factor in chronic ligament instability of the ankle. *Foot Ankle Int* 1997;18:402–405.

6. Myerson M (ed): *Current Therapy in Foot and Ankle Surgery.* St. Louis, MO, Mosby-Yearbook, 1993, pp 203–209.

7. Scranton PE, McDermott JE, Rogers JV: The relationship between chronic ankle instability and variation in mortise anatomy and impingement spurs. *Foot Ankle,* in press.

8. Bröstrom L: Sprained ankles: VI. Surgical treatment of "chronic" ligament ruptures. *Acta Chir Scand* 1966;132:551–565.

9. Gould N, Seligson D, Gassman J: Early and late repair of lateral ligament of the ankle. *Foot Ankle* 1980;1:84–89.

10. Hamilton WG, Thompson FM, Snow SW: The modified Bröstrom procedure for lateral ankle instability. *Foot Ankle* 1993;14:1–7.

11. Scranton PE Jr, McDermott JE: Anterior tibiotalar spurs: A comparison of open versus arthroscopic debridement. *Foot Ankle* 1992;13:125–129.

12. Sammarco GJ, DiRaimondo CV: Surgical treatment of lateral ankle instability syndrome. *Am J Sports Med* 1988;16:501–511.

13. Snook GA, Chrisman OD, Wilson TC: Long-term results of the Chrisman-Snook operation for reconstruction of the lateral ligaments of the ankle. *J Bone Joint Surg* 1985;67A:1–7.

14. Sarrafian SK (ed): *Anatomy of the Foot and Ankle: Descriptive, Topographic, Functional.* Philadelphia, PA, JB Lippincott, 1983.

15. Sobel M, Mizel MS: Peroneal tendon injury, in Pfeffer GB, Frey CC (eds): *Current Practice in Foot and Ankle Surgery.* New York, NY, McGraw-Hill, Health Professions Division, 1993, pp 30–56.

16. McMaster JH, Scranton PE Jr: Tibiofibular synostosis: A cause of ankle disability. *Clin Orthop* 1975;111:172–174.

17. Kollias SL, Ferkel RD: Fibular grooving for recurrent peroneal tendon subluxation. *Am J Sports Med* 1997;25:329–335.

# INJURIES TO THE SUBTALAR JOINT

## CAROL FREY, MD

## INTRODUCTION

It is not unusual for the subtalar joint to be injured after an inversion injury to the ankle joint. During the workup of an athlete with an ankle sprain or chronic pain and/or instability, the differential diagnosis of pathology in the subtalar joint should be considered. This chapter will review diagnoses that can occur after an ankle sprain.

A careful history and physical examination may point to the subtalar joint as the focus of the injury. The first indication of an injury to the subtalar joint after an ankle sprain may be Battle's sign, ecchymosis that develops over the medial border of the hindfoot (Fig. 1). However, the complex anatomy of the subtalar joint often makes radiographic and physical examination difficult. A better understanding of the anatomy of the hindfoot, and the subtalar joint in particular, will greatly facilitate the diagnostic workup, physical examination, performance of surgery, and proper recognition of abnormal pathology when it is present.

## ANATOMY

The subtalar joint can be divided into anterior and posterior sections by the sinus tarsi and the tarsal canal (Fig. 2, *A*). Contents of the tarsal canal include the cervical ligament, talocalcaneal interosseous ligament, medial root of the inferior extensor retinaculum, fat pad, and blood vessels (Fig. 2, *B*). The anterior portion of the subtalar joint, also known as the talocalcaneonavicular joint, includes the anteri-

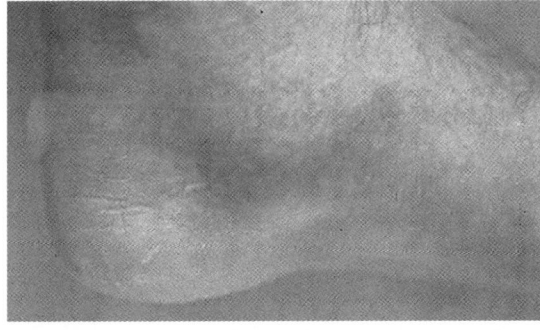

**FIGURE 1**
"Battle's sign." Ecchymosis on the medial aspect of the hindfoot, indicating an injury to the subtalar joint.

or and middle articulating facets, the talonavicular articulation, and the spring ligament. The anterior subtalar joint is separated from the posterior subtalar joint by the thick interosseous ligament, which fills the tarsal canal.

The posterior subtalar joint has a long axis that is located obliquely 40° to the midline of the foot and faces laterally. It consists of the convex posterior facet of the calcaneus and the concave posterior facet of the talus. The capsule of the posterior subtalar joint is reinforced laterally by the cervical, calcaneofibular, and lateral talocalcaneal ligaments and has a posterior pouch and a small lateral recess.

## BIOMECHANICS

The basic motion of the subtalar joint has been described as that of eversion and inversion.[1,2] Range of motion of the subtalar joint is tested by holding the left heel in the right hand or vice versa, then using the opposite hand to grasp the

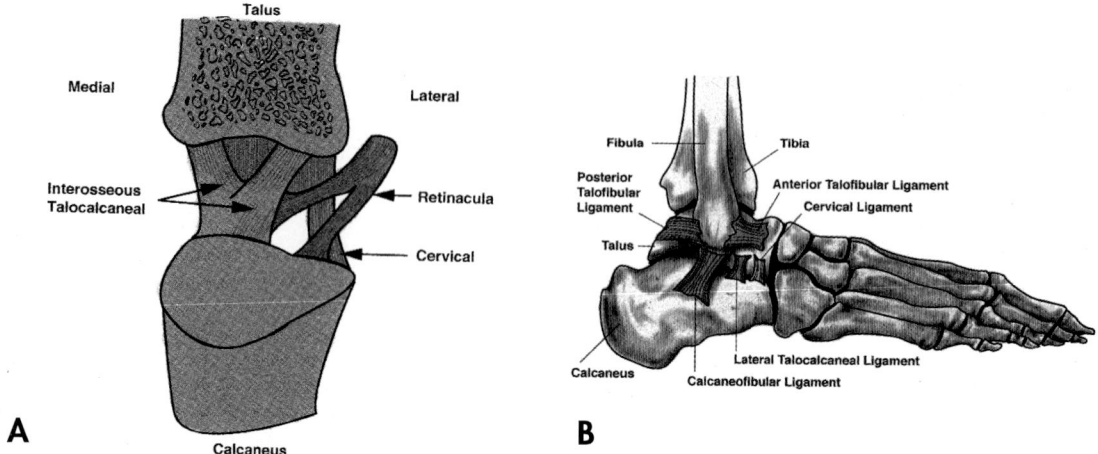

**FIGURE 2**
**A,** The subtalar joint can be divided into anterior and posterior sections by the sinus tarsi, the tarsal canal, and its contents. **B,** The contents of the tarsal canal include the cervical ligament, talocalcaneal interosseous ligament, medial root of the inferior extensor retinaculum, fat pad, and blood vessels.

forefoot and move the heel from inversion to eversion. The motion should be pain-free and smooth. Although there is a variable degree of subtalar motion, it usually is 24°.[3]

Range of motion of the subtalar joint is linked with motion in the ankle joint. External rotation at the ankle causes the subtalar joint to become more perpendicular to the walking surface and increases subtalar motion. As the foot internally rotates, the ankle joint becomes more perpendicular to the floor and decreases motion at the subtalar joint.

## RADIOGRAPHIC EXAMINATION

The subtalar joint is difficult to examine radiographically. The anterior portion of the subtalar joint is best seen on a 45° lateral oblique view of the foot. The posterior facet of the joint is best seen on a Broden view, which is taken with the foot in dorsiflexion and medially rotated 45°. The X-ray beam is angled 10° cephalad and directed at the lateral malleolus. The angle of the x-ray beam increases from 10° to 40° to obtain the different Broden views of the subtalar joint. Computed tomography (CT) scans show intra-articular and bone pathology and have replaced plain tomography. CT is recommended particularly in the evaluation of fractures and tarsal coalitions.

Magnetic resonance imaging (MRI) has been useful in studying the soft tissues around the ankle joint and hindfoot. The anatomy of the foot and ankle is complex and lends itself well to multiplanar imaging. In my own series of patients who have suffered injuries to the subtalar joint after an ankle sprain, several diagnoses have been made with MRI, including interosseous ligament tears, arthrofibrosis, and ganglion cysts.

No one test stands out as the best in the evaluation of subtalar instability. Stress radiographs, arthrograms, and stress tomograms are limited by the fact that normal subtalar motion has not been well defined.[3–7] The most practical test to obtain in an orthopaedic office is a standard stress test of the ankle joint that includes the subtalar joint. Clanton[5] points out that loss of parallelism of the facets of the posterior subtalar joint with the varus stress test will occur with subtalar instability. Anterior subluxation of the calcaneus with respect to the talus with the anterior drawer test also indicates subtalar instability. More normal subtalar joints need to be assessed before a clear recommendation can be made in the radiographic evaluation of subtalar instability.

# FRACTURES

## LATERAL PROCESS OF THE TALUS

Extending from the lower margin of the talar articular surface of the fibula to the posteroinferior surface of the talus is the lateral process of the talus. It is wedge shaped and consists of a varied amount of the lateral aspect of the talar body. The process has an articular and a nonarticular surface. Its articular surface is the most lateral part of the posteroinferior joint surface of the talus. The lateral process serves as an insertion site for the lateral talocalcaneal, cervical, and anterior talofibular ligaments and can be injured after an inversion sprain. The talofibular articulation of the ankle joint and the posterior talocalcaneal articulation of the subtalar joint may be involved in a fracture of the lateral process of the talus, depending on the size of the fracture fragment.

A fracture of the lateral process of the talus has a very similar history and clinical findings to an injury of the lateral collateral ligaments of the ankle. It usually occurs in a young male who has fallen from a height, suffered a snowboarding accident, stepped into a hole, or has been involved in a motor vehicle accident. The history is almost identical to that of an ankle sprain, with immediate swelling and localized pain and tenderness over the lateral process of the talus. Rarely is crepitus present. The pain will increase with dorsiflexion and plantarflexion movement at the ankle and inversion or eversion at the subtalar joint. This injury is easily misdiagnosed as just an ankle sprain.

Radiographic examination should begin with a routine foot and ankle series. If the lateral process and the sustentaculum tali do not overlap, the lateral view is the most helpful in evaluating the fracture. The anteroposterior (AP) view, with the ankle in neutral and the leg internally rotated 20°, can also show the fracture. In suspicious cases, an oblique radiograph of the ankle with the foot in 45° of internal rotation and 30° of equinus is recommended. When evaluating the radiographs, note that a normal accessory ossicle may occur in the area of the lateral process of the talus. A bone scan is recommended to evaluate suspicious cases, and a high resolution CT scan to assess fracture size, location, presence, and amount of displacement.

Dorsiflexion and inversion of the foot is probably the most common mechanism of fracture of the lateral process. The articular surfaces of the posterior subtalar joint are congruous with weightbearing but when the heel is inverted, the head of the talus slides laterally and the posterior subtalar joint becomes incongruous. When the foot is in the inverted position, acute dorsiflexion forces concentrate on the lateral process of the talus. A fracture can result from the compression forces on the lateral process of the talus. Other associated injuries that may occur with dorsiflexion and inversion are fractures of the talar neck, anterior subtalar dislocations, adduction type fractures of the medial malleolus, avulsion fracture of the lateral malleolus, and complete ruptures of the lateral collateral ligaments.

Studies of snowboarding injuries indicate that lateral process fractures are associated with higher levels of expertise and the use of older soft-shell boots.[8] In addition, aerial maneuvers and jumps, which cause the athlete to land with the feet in forced dorsiflexion and inversion, can lead to the injury.

A type I fracture of the lateral process has been described as a chip fracture of the anteroinferior aspect.[9,10] This fracture does not extend into the joint and may represent an avulsion fracture of the anterior talofibular ligament. Type II is a simple fracture with a large fragment, usually nondisplaced and extending from the talofibular joint surface to the posterior subtalar joint surface. Type II is subdivided into IIA, a nondisplaced single large fragment, and IIB, a displaced single large fragment. Type III involves a comminuted fracture of both the fibular and posterior subtalar articular surfaces and may involve the entire lateral process.[10]

Treatment depends on the amount of displacement, the size of the fracture fragment, the degree of comminution, and the compression of articular cartilage. Closed treatment is most successful in acute nondisplaced fractures and when an acceptable reduction can be obtained. With the foot in a neutral or an everted position, the lateral process may be manipulated into position and a short leg nonweightbearing cast applied for 4 weeks. A posterior splint and range-of-motion exercises follow this.

A displaced fracture of greater than 1.5 cm may require open reduction and internal fixation with a compression screw. A Herbert screw works well in this location. Immobilization is then carried out with a short leg nonweightbearing cast. At 4 weeks, a posterior splint and range-of-motion exercises are recommended until there is radiographic healing. Radiographic healing may occur around 6 weeks. Weightbearing is begun at 4 to 6 weeks.

A comminuted fracture of less than 1.5 cm or one that has significant cartilage damage should be excised. Excision allows for early range of motion and weightbearing.

Even with adequate initial treatment, pain with weightbearing is the most common long-term sequela after fractures to the lateral process.[11] Hawkins[9] reported weightbearing pain, which resulted in surgical exploration in 50% of his patients. He also reported that a symptomatic nonunion of the lateral process was not uncommon. Other long-term problems include bone overgrowth and impingement in the sinus tarsi or talofibular joint. Problems may develop with osteoarthritis, nonunion, malalignment, and osseous overgrowth. A patient who develops these will have chronic pain and limitation of subtalar motion and ankle dorsiflexion. Poor results are more common in cases that are diagnosed late. Excision of the fragment or subtalar fusion may be indicated to treat a symptomatic nonunion, malunion, or overgrowth and impingement of bone.

## ANTERIOR PROCESS OF THE CALCANEUS

Fractures of the anterior process of the calcaneus are avulsion injuries. This fracture may be overlooked initially, especially after an inversion injury to the ankle. The incidence of these fractures has been reported as anywhere from 3% to 23% of fractures of the calcaneus.[12–21]

The anterior aspect of the calcaneus has been referred to by a variety of terms including the anterior process, anterior lip, anterosuperior portion, anterosuperior process, promontory, and the anterior end of the calcaneus. This area of the calcaneus can be a large beak-shaped prominence that overhangs the calcaneocuboid joint or it can be a small eminence. Articular cartilage may exist on a large prominence that may articulate with the talus or the cuboid.

The lateral aspect of the anterior calcaneal process is the origin of the bifurcate ligament, which attaches distally to the navicular and cuboid bones. The extensor digitorum brevis muscle may also have a small area of origin from the anterior process.

The most common mechanism of fracture of the anterior process is following an inversion-plantarflexion injury. The anterior process is avulsed by the bifurcate ligament. This may occur in conjunction with an injury to the lateral collateral ligaments of the ankle. If the ankle has suffered a sprain to the lateral collateral ligaments at the same time as a fracture to the anterior process, the fracture diagnosis may be overlooked.

When the hindfoot is fixed, a compression fracture of the anterior process may occur with dorsiflexion and forced abduction of the forefoot. Compared to an avulsion injury, this fracture may be more commonly displaced and associated with an injury to the calcaneocuboid joint.

Regardless of the mechanism, when a fracture of the anterior process occurs, the athlete may feel a pop or crack. The patient reports pain over the anterior process of the calcaneus at the lateral border of the foot. The pain will usually increase with weightbearing activities.

The physical examination reveals tenderness on palpation over the anterior process of the calcaneus. Range of motion of the subtalar joint will usually increase the pain. In acute cases, swelling and ecchymosis may also be present. Spasms and guarding from the peroneal muscles may be present after the fracture.

An oblique radiograph of the foot taken with the central beam directed 15° to 20° superior and posterior to the midfoot is the best view to detect these fractures (Fig. 3). The AP and lateral views of the foot may not reveal an injury, and the diagnosis may be missed. An accessory ossicle can occur in this location and should be ruled out during the evaluation of a patient with a possible fracture of the anterior process. This ossicle, known as the calcaneus secundaris, has the typical rounded smooth cortical margins of an ossicle. An acute fracture will have irregular margins and typically will have a triangular shape. A nonunion will also appear triangular, but with sclerotic margins. Radiographs should be examined for the size of the fracture fragment, degree of displacement, and involvement of the anterior subtalar facet or calcaneocuboid articulation.

In general, the major concern with fractures of the anterior process is a delay in diagnosis. If treated early, fractures of the anterior process of the calcaneus usually take 2 to 3 months to unite, but the patient may not be completely free of symptoms for up to a year. Optimizing function of the subtalar joint takes precedence over an anatomic union.

If the fracture fragment is small, minimally displaced, and does not involve a joint surface, the prognosis is good. With nonsurgical treatment of these fractures, Degan and associates[16] reported good results with no long-term activity limitations. However, the average time to recovery in this series was 10 months. For small nondisplaced fractures with minimal joint involvement, the foot is placed in a short leg removable cast or fracture boot with elevation and compression. At 5 to 7 days, after the inflammatory phase, the patient removes the cast 3 to 4 times a day for range-of-motion exercises. In addition, range of motion of the toes is recommended to decrease edema in the foot. The patient is nonweightbearing for 2 to 4 weeks and then allowed to bear weight as tolerated. The removable cast or boot may be permanently removed when the fracture is clinically healed.

If the fracture is 1.5 cm or larger and displaced, or involves a significant amount of joint surface, an open reduction and internal fixation is recommended. The patient is placed into a posterior splint. Range-of-motion exercises and weight-

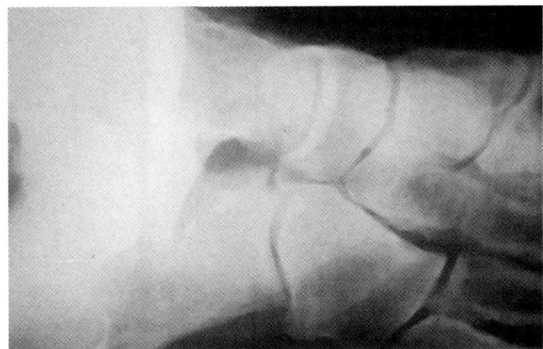

**FIGURE 3**
A fracture of the anterior process of the calcaneus.

bearing begin after the wound has healed and inflammation significantly decreased.

If a painful nonunion occurs, excision of the fragment is recommended. After the inflammatory period has passed, weightbearing and range-of-motion exercises begin. However, even after the excision, recovery may be prolonged, and it may take up to 1 year for the patient to be completely free of symptoms. If the patient remains symptomatic after excision of the fragment, an arthrodesis of the subtalar joint or the calcaneocuboid joint, whichever is determined to be symptomatic, may have to be performed.

## POSTERIOR PROCESS OF THE TALUS

The posterior surface of the talus, or "processus posterior tali," consists of both the posteromedial and posterolateral processes, also known as tubercles (Fig. 4). The posterior process and its tubercles can vary in size and shape. The flexor hallucis longus (FHL) glides in a sulcus between the 2 tubercles.[22] The larger posterolateral process, also called Stieda's process, can vary markedly in size. It is in direct continuity inferiorly with the posterolateral aspect of the articular surface of the talus, making it a partially intra-articular structure. Its superior surface, however, is nonarticular, because it is part of the insertion of the posterior talofibular ligament. Occasionally, an accessory ossicle can communicate with the posterolateral tubercle, and this is called the os trigonum. It too has multiple surfaces—anterior, inferior, and posterior. The former 2 articulate with the posterolat-

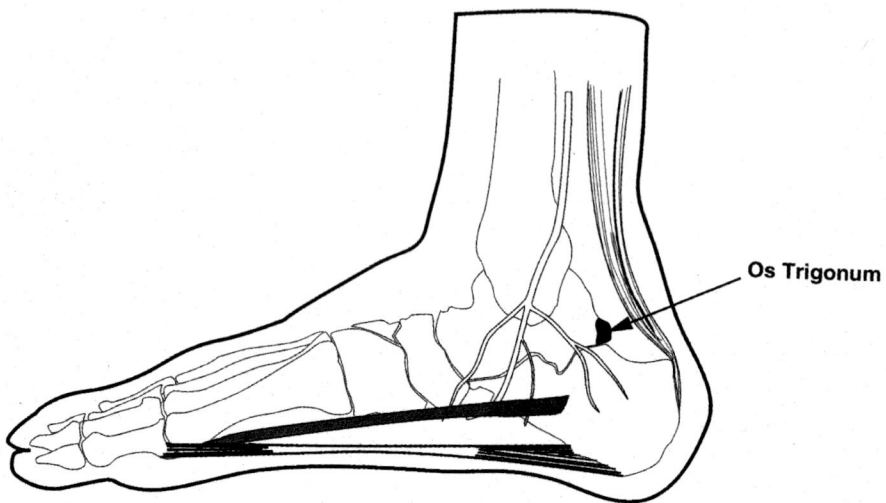

**FIGURE 4**
Anatomy of Stieda's process and the os trigonum.

eral tubercle or os calcis, respectively, and the latter is nonarticular. It often is difficult to discern a fracture of Stieda's process from an os trigonum based on radiographs alone. Use of a technetium 99m bone scan, a CT scan, and views of the opposite foot can be helpful.

## OS TRIGONUM

The os trigonum and trigonal process are normal structures that do not create symptoms for most people. The structures may become symptomatic after activities that require extreme plantarflexion or after trauma. After an injury, the bony structures or the adjacent soft tissues may be damaged. In 1882, Shepherd[23] reported that the os trigonum was not an accessory bone but a fractured posterolateral process of the talus. A previously intact process may be fractured as a result of the compression forces generated during plantarflexion. Cadaver studies show that the posterior talofibular ligaments and posterior talocalcaneal ligaments can displace a fractured trigonal process, a mechanism that may occur with an avulsion injury. Once injured, the posterior structure may act as a block to full plantarflexion.

More than 50% of patients attribute their condition to an athletic or work-related injury. Paulos and associates[24] reported that 20 patients with persistent posterior ankle pain after a previous ankle sprain were found to have posterior talar process injuries. They also reported that 50% of their patients with posterior talar process fractures responded to conservative treatment. The acute injuries did well in all cases, but the majority of the chronic cases did poorly.

Forced plantarflexion of the foot can cause a direct impact with the posterior tibial plafond, which fractures the posterior process of the talus or the syndesmosis of the os trigonum. Subsequent distracting forces from ligament attachment sites can lead to the development of a painful nonunion. A large posterior process can fracture, the os trigonum may remain intact but become symptomatic, and the os trigonum can separate at the synchondrosis.

Initial treatment of the fracture includes a short leg walking cast until the patient is clinically healed, usually at 4 to 6 weeks. This is followed by range-of-motion exercises that avoid forced plantarflexion for 12 weeks.

Excision is recommended if the posterior lateral process or the os trigonum continues to be symptomatic despite conservative treatment. Open and arthroscopic techniques have been reported for surgical excision of the injured structure. Hamilton[25] informs his patients that it takes 3 to 8 months for full recovery following open excision. Other authors[26,27] reported that full recovery may take even longer, with 5 to 12 months of recovery common. However, all of the arthroscopic patients reported in Ferkel's series[27] were functioning at 3 months after the operation. With improved recovery time and low morbidity, arthroscopic excision may have an advantage over open excision.

Hamilton[25] noted in his series of classical ballet dancers, that a stenosing tenosynovitis of the FHL was commonly found in association with an injury to the posterolateral process or os trigonum. A tenolysis of the FHL tendon was required in 15 of 17 feet undergoing an excision of an os trigonum in Hamilton's group of patients. Brodsky and Khalil[28] did not note any pathology of the FHL. In his series of patients treated arthroscopically, Ferkel[27] reported only 1 injury to the FHL.

Arthroscopic excision of the os trigonum has been reported to be a good alternative to open treatment for patients who require surgical intervention. Compared to open incisions, properly placed arthroscopic portals offer a decreased risk of skin necrosis, incisional neuromas, and cutaneous scarring.

Subtalar arthroscopy using standard portals is performed first (Fig. 5). The borders of the os trigonum are carefully identified using small-joint instruments such as a full radius shaver and probe. Care must be taken when working near the posterior and medial borders of the os trigonum to avoid injury to the FHL and posterior tibial neurovascular bundle. When free of soft-tissue attachment, the os trigonum is delivered with a grasper through an enlarged posterior portal. An accessory posterior subtalar portal may occasionally be required under these circumstances. FHL pathology may not be treated arthroscopically.

## OCCULT FRACTURES

Osteochondral lesions of the talus are not limited to the dome. They may also involve the subtalar joint and the talonavicular joint. The talus is covered with cartilage over two thirds of its surface

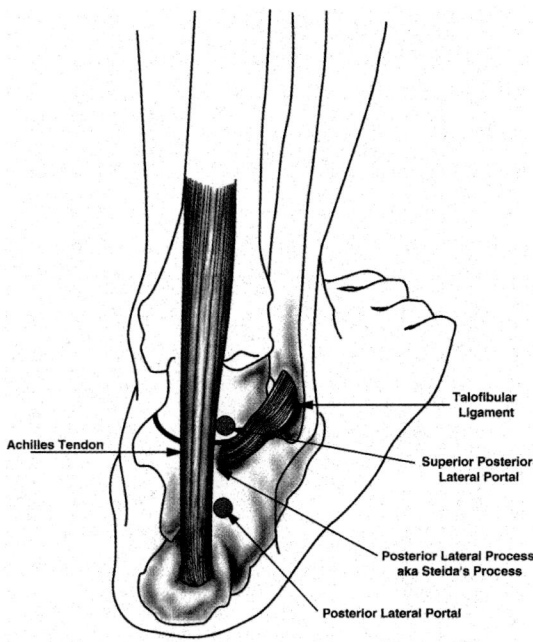

**FIGURE 5**
Portals used for arthroscopic resection of the os trigonum.

and has 7 different weightbearing surfaces. Osteochondral fractures may occur with any trauma applied across the articular surfaces, and any of the surfaces may be injured after an ankle sprain.

Osteochondral lesions of the inferior talus are often missed and can be a cause of persistent symptoms of pain, crepitus, and limitation of subtalar motion after an ankle sprain. The initial injury is often treated as "just a sprain."

A bone scan is the best screening test to evaluate a patient for osteochondral lesions of the talus. Bone scans were able to identify fractures in all cases presented in a study by Burkus and associates.[29] Even so, the diagnosis was delayed an average of 11 months for the patients in this series.

The recommended treatment for nondisplaced acute injuries is casting. If symptoms persist or the lesion is displaced, surgical treatment is recommended. Surgical options include excision of the lesion, retrograde drilling, antegrade drilling, or abrasion of the lesion. The decision-making process is similar to that for osteochondral lesions of the ankle. The lesions may be approached through an open incision or with arthroscopic techniques.

## SUBTALAR DISLOCATIONS

Subtalar dislocations are uncommon athletic injuries that involve a dislocation of the talonavicular joint and talocalcaneal joint. Medial dislocations of the subtalar joint are more common after an inversion injury and are more frequent than lateral dislocations. Simple inversion injuries, which result in a medial subtalar dislocation, have been referred to as "basketball foot" because these injuries occur most commonly while playing this sport. Lateral dislocation requires more energy to produce and has more fractures associated with it.[30] Early motion of the subtalar joint should be initiated as soon as possible after a dislocation. Open reduction and internal fixation of an associated fracture may facilitate early range of motion.

After this injury, most patients will return to activities but may note a limp or pain when walking on uneven ground. At least 80% of patients with this injury will have some restriction of subtalar motion in the long run, and the majority of patients will develop subtalar arthritis. If intra-articular fractures are associated with the dislocation, the chance of degenerative changes occurring is higher. With an inversion injury, the sustentaculum tali acts as a fulcrum on the posterior part of the talus, which can result in medial dislocation. The dislocation is believed to occur first at the talonavicular joint. The forces continue through the rest of the subtalar joint complex as a complete dislocation of the subtalar joint occurs. Poor results are believed to be linked to associated fractures, soft-tissue injury, and prolonged immobilization.

## SUBTALAR INSTABILITY

Subtalar instability after inversion injuries to the ankle is probably a lot more common than reported. The instability can have characteristics of chronic lateral instability or recurrent ankle sprains. Subtalar instability remains poorly defined, although it has been described by several authors. Instability of the subtalar joint is difficult to diagnose and treat.[3-7] It is difficult to evaluate clinically and radiographically. Although it is most commonly associated with ankle instability, subtalar instability can exist on its own.

Harper[31] has divided the lateral ligaments of the subtalar joint into the superficial, intermediate, and deep layers. The superficial layer includes the lateral limb of the inferior extensor retinaculum, the lateral talocalcaneal ligament, and the calcaneofibular ligament. The intermediate layer includes the intermediate root of the inferior extensor retinaculum, which inserts on the floor of the sinus tarsi, and the cervical ligament. The deep layer includes the medial root of the inferior extensor retinaculum and the interosseous talocalcaneal ligament, which fills the tarsal canal.

Tears of the ligaments of the subtalar joint are caused by supination injuries to the ankle and the hindfoot. The calcaneofibular, lateral talocalcaneal, cervical, and interosseous talocalcaneal ligaments are subjected to injury in that order.[3] Subtalar joint injuries are divided into 4 types of injury mechanics and ligament damage.[3] Type I injuries are from a forced supination of the hindfoot, associated with either plantarflexion or dorsiflexion of the ankle. With the plantarflexed ankle, the anterior talofibular ligament of the ankle may be injured. In the subtalar joint, the cervical ligament is torn first followed by disruption of the calcaneofibular ligament and the lateral capsule. In a type II injury, in addition to the above injuries, rupture of the interosseous talocalcaneal ligament occurs. With the ankle in dorsiflexion, type III injuries can occur with severe soft-tissue injury to the calcaneofibular, cervical, and interosseous talocalcaneal ligaments. The anterior talofibular ligament remains intact with this injury. Type IV injury includes severe damage to the ankle and subtalar ligaments. This injury is produced by forceful supination of the hindfoot with the ankle initially in dorsiflexion and subsequently moving into plantarflexion.

Pipkin[32] described a mechanism of injury to the interosseous talocalcaneal ligament that occurs in triple jumpers and basketball players. In these athletes, the abrupt impact and deceleration of the calcaneus with the talus continuing to move forward from inertia results in injury to the subtalar joint. This has been described as a "whiplash" mechanism of injury to the interosseous ligaments of the subtalar joint.

Patients with chronic subtalar instability typically have symptoms of giving way and a history of recurrent sprains. The true incidence of these injuries is not known. It is assumed that most subtalar joint injuries occur along with injuries to the lateral collateral ligaments of the ankle, and the incidence has been thought to be as high as 25% of those who suffer from chronic ankle instability.[6]

Clinical evaluation of the patient with subtalar instability is difficult. The symptoms may include tenderness over the sinus tarsi or deep pain in the subtalar joint. More than varus instability, the patient with subtalar instability will demonstrate increased internal rotation of the calcaneus on physical examination when stress is applied. The patient with subtalar instability may also demonstrate increased distal displacement of the calcaneus in relation to the talus as compared to the uninjured side.

One of the major problems in the diagnosis of subtalar instability is the lack of consensus as to a definition. Authors have reported on subtalar stress views, subtalar arthrography, and stress tomogram to define instability. Brantigan and associates[4] recommended a tomographic stress test to evaluate instability of the subtalar joint. Heilman and associates[33] suggested a Broden stress view for evaluating subtalar instability. Clanton[5] also recommends a 40° Broden stress view.

In the normal subtalar joint, subtalar arthrograms will demonstrate radiographic dye moving freely within the joint. After an acute injury to the subtalar joint, an arthrogram may be performed by placing the syringe into the posterior joint and injecting radiopaque dye. Injury is confirmed if there is leakage of the contrast material into the ankle joint, surrounding soft tissues, or the sinus tarsi. In the case of chronic injury to the ligaments of the subtalar joint, the lateral recess of the joint may not fill with dye. In addition, at the anterior aspect of the posterior subtalar joint there may be a blunt appearance of the dye, and the normal small recess along the talocalcaneal ligament will not be present. None of these methods, however, have gained clinical acceptance in the evaluation of subtalar joint instability because their diagnostic accuracy has not been demonstrated.

Karlsson and associates[3] used standard stress radiographs of the ankle joint to include the subtalar joint in the views. In the normal joint there is close congruity of the articular surfaces of the talus and the calcaneus. Subtalar joint instability is defined as separation of the joint surface of greater than or equal to 2 mm in the AP view as compared to the normal side. Laurin and associates[34] note that any loss of parallelism between the talus and calcaneus is diagnostic of instability of the subtalar joint when viewing standard stress radiographs of the ankle joint under varus stress. Heilman and associates[33] reported separation of ≥ 5 mm between the joint surfaces on the AP view as diagnostic. During the anterior drawer test, the calcaneus may be seen to slide anterior with respect to the talus, indicating subtalar instability.[35]

Even though stress views and Broden views make it possible to view the subtalar joint better, there is still a problem in that normal values for talocalcaneal motion and displacement have never been well defined. A standard stress view, taken as a Broden projection at 45°, may allow better distinction between subtalar and ankle instability.[3] The normally parallel posterior facets of the subtalar joint are seen clearly on this view.

Direct observation of the joint may be the most accurate way of evaluating the unstable joint. When varus stress is applied to the subtalar joint at the time of arthroscopy, the posterior calcaneal facet glides medially out from under the talus[36] (Fig. 6). This may represent one part of the screw-like motion of the subtalar joint.[1,2,37] Further experience with observing normal motion of the subtalar joint during arthroscopy should lead to greater confidence in recommending arthroscopic stress tests in the evaluation of subtalar instability.

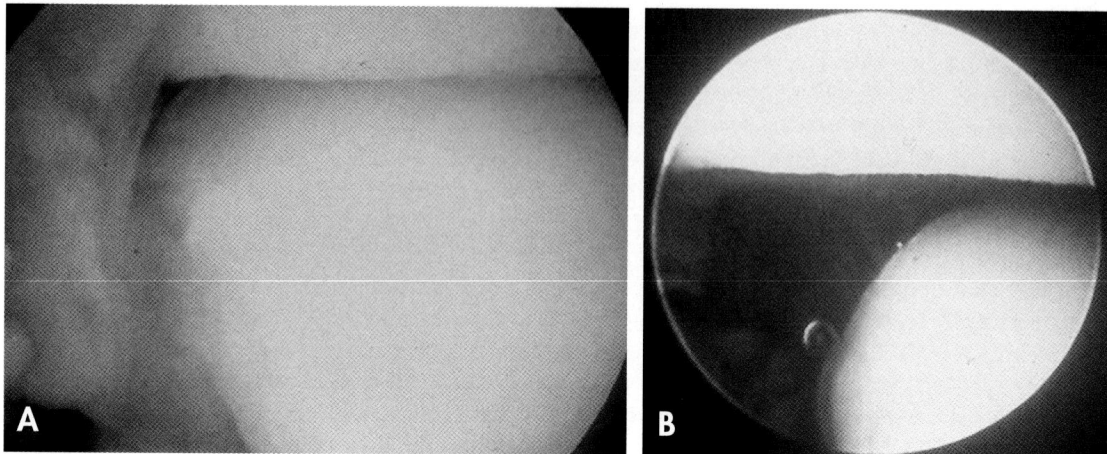

**FIGURE 6**
Instability of the subtalar joint demonstrated at arthroscopy. **A,** The lateral aspect of the posterior subtalar joint before varus stress. **B,** The joint after varus stress. The calcaneus glides medially under the talus.

Treatment of subtalar instability is similar to that of chronic ankle instability. Nonsurgical treatment includes peroneal strengthening, Achilles tendon stretching, and proprioceptive exercises. A brace may be used that includes a hindfoot lock to stabilize the subtalar joint, and taping should include a heel lock. Other treatment methods include a lateral heel wedge or a University of California Berkeley (UCB) orthosis to decrease excursion of the subtalar joint. Most patients will respond well to nonsurgical treatment.

A direct repair of the ligaments or a tendon transfer are recommended for chronic subtalar instability. One example of a tendon transfer, which will correct subtalar instability, is the Larsen[38] procedure (Fig. 7). In this procedure, the tendon of the peroneus brevis is transferred through drill holes in the fibula, under the peroneal tendons, and into the calcaneus. A suture, a staple, or a suture fixation device may anchor the tendon. Although this procedure was originally recommended using the entire peroneus brevis, the tendon may be split for the procedure.

Chrisman and Snook[39] reported that 3 of 7 patients they investigated who had ankle instability had concurrent subtalar instability. Because their modification of the Elmslie procedure is designed to reconstruct both the anterior talofibular ligament and the calcaneofibular ligament, it can be used to treat instability of the ankle and subtalar joint. As expected, the operation restricts motion in the subtalar joint. The modified Elmslie repair, or Chrisman-Snook procedure, involves splitting the peroneus brevis tendon and passing it through a bone tunnel in the fibula, through a

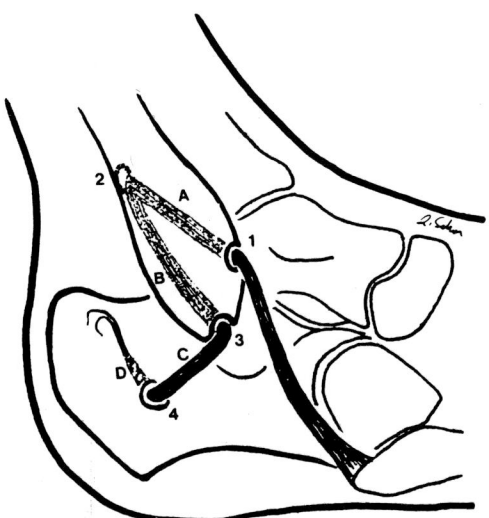

**FIGURE 7**
Ligament repairs for subtalar instability using the peroneal tendons. (Reproduced with permission from Schon LC, Clanton TO, Baxter DE: Reconstruction for subtalar instability: A review. *Foot Ankle* 1991;11:319–325.)

tunnel on the lateral side of the calcaneus, and then suturing the tendon back onto itself. Chrisman and Snook[39] modified the procedure to pass the posterior limb of the tendon graft over the top of the peroneal tendons to decrease the incidence of tendon subluxation. The surgeon must take care not to suture this limb too tightly and entrap the tendons underneath the graft. Because the remaining limb of the peroneus brevis will hypertrophy with time, the patient sacrifices little or no peroneal function when this tendon transfer is used.

A triligament reconstruction has been recommended that uses the plantaris tendon[7] (Fig. 8). The isolated plantaris tendon should measure 32 to 34 cm to adequately perform the repair. The starting point for the first bone tunnel is at the attachment site of the calcaneofibular ligament. The bone tunnels in the fibula are created approximately 2 cm proximal to the distal tip of the fibula and 2 cm posterior to the anterior border of the fibula. Another tunnel is made from the anterosuperior border of the anterior talofibular ligament and is directed toward the hole, which is 2 cm proximal to the distal tip of the fibula. A V-shaped tunnel in the lateral talus and a final lateral calcaneal tunnel, just under Gissane's angle, are created. A 3.5-mm drill bit is used to create the bone tunnels. The graft is then passed from the medial aspect of the calcaneus, under the peroneal tendons, through the fibula, talus, and calcaneus and then back the same route until the tendon is sutured to the tissues along the posteromedial aspect of the calcaneus or to itself. It is sometimes difficult to find a plantaris tendon of sufficient length and strength. In that case, a split peroneus brevis tendon graft may be used as a substitute in this reconstruction. If the plantaris tendon is used, the procedure does not compromise function of the peroneal tendons and provides a near anatomic reconstruction of the anterior talofibular, calcaneofibular, and cervical ligaments. Furthermore, there is no restriction of motion in either the ankle or the subtalar joint after this procedure. The triligament reconstruction addresses both ankle and subtalar instability. Comparative studies reported in the literature indicate that this repair is best.[7]

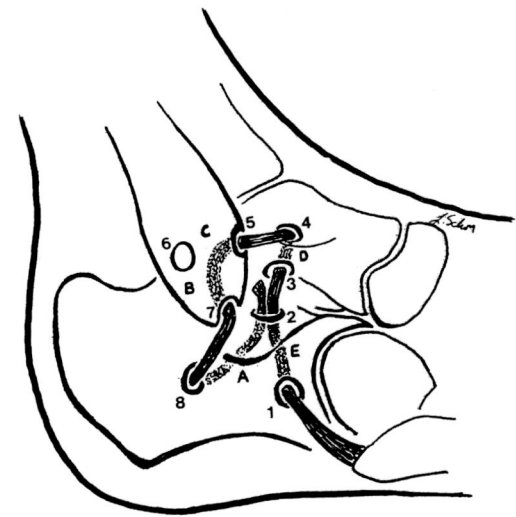

**FIGURE 8**
Triligament repair for subtalar instability. (Reproduced with permission from Schon LC, Clanton TO, Baxter DE: Reconstruction for subtalar instability: A review. *Foot Ankle* 1991;11:319–325.)

The inferior extensor retinaculum reinforcement of the Bröstrom procedure, as described by Gould,[40] can be used in patients with combined instability. Because the calcaneofibular ligament is repaired and the inferior extensor retinaculum attaches to the floor of the sinus tarsi, the subtalar joint is stabilized with this procedure (Fig. 9).

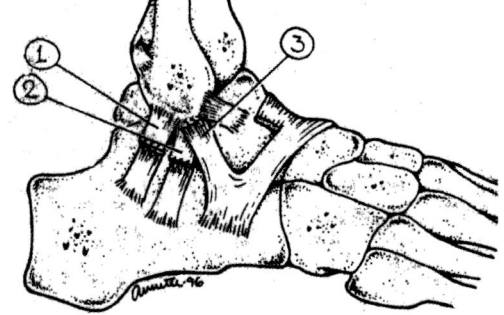

**FIGURE 9**
Anatomic repair of the calcaneofibular, lateral talocalcaneal, and cervical ligaments. The repair is augmented with the inferior extensor retinaculum. (Reproduced with permission from Karlsson J, Eriksson BI, Renstrom P: Subtalar instability of the foot. *Scand J Med Sci Sports* 1998;8:191–197.)

## TALAR COALITION

Tarsal coalition is a bridging between the tarsal bones of the foot. The bridge may be composed of bone, cartilage, fibrous tissue, or a combination of these. The coalition may be complete or incomplete. The incidence of tarsal coalition is less than 1% of the general population, and the most common types bridge the talocalcaneal and calcaneonavicular joints. Tarsal coalitions are thought to be secondary to a failure of segmentation and differentiation of the primitive mesenchyme. The terms ossified, nonossified, and partially ossified have also been used to describe tarsal coalition. When symptomatic, patients commonly complain of hindfoot pain and have a history of frequent ankle sprains. A tarsal coalition should be ruled out in an individual who suffers from frequent inversion injuries to the ankle. Furthermore, a previously asymptomatic coalition may become symptomatic after an injury such as an ankle sprain.

The most common symptom of a tarsal coalition among athletes, adolescents, and young adults is repeat ankle sprains. Chronic pain may persist after the sprain. For talonavicular coalition, ossification occurs when patients are between 3 and 5 years old. For calcaneonavicular coalition, ossification occurs between 8 and 12 years, and for talocalcaneal coalition between 12 and 16 years. At birth and in early childhood, the coalition is fibrous or cartilaginous. Some motion occurs between the bones involved in the coalition, and the foot is asymptomatic. As the coalition ossifies, subtalar motion is restricted and the foot becomes symptomatic; frequently this occurs after an ankle sprain. Scranton[41] noted that the coalition can become symptomatic in adults after trauma.

The classic appearance is a rigid flatfoot with heel valgus and abduction of the forefoot. The heel usually has a valgus deformity but may be in neutral or varus. With tarsal coalition, normal inversion-eversion of the subtalar joint is absent or severely limited. Compensatory motion must occur in the ankle joint or distal to the subtalar joint, causing progressive laxity. The forefoot is abducted, the arch flattens, and the navicular bone overrides the talus, which often leads to talar beaking.

On physical examination, the calcaneonavicular coalition is usually painful directly over the coalition at the sinus tarsi. The talocalcaneal coalition may be painful over the medial talocalcaneal joint, but usually the pain is present deep in the subtalar joint, and often it is poorly localized. A prominent coalition of the middle facet may cause some impingement of the contents of the tarsal tunnel, with resultant pain and numbness.

Talocalcaneal coalitions usually eliminate subtalar motion, and are more likely than other coalitions to produce a severe valgus hindfoot. Patients with calcaneonavicular coalitions usually have a valgus hindfoot and loss of subtalar motion, but to a lesser degree than with a talocalcaneal coalition.

The radiographic evaluation of a patient with suspected tarsal coalition should include a standard foot series with axial hindfoot views as described by Harris.[42] For the diagnosis of a calcaneonavicular bar, a 45° lateral oblique view of the foot is the best. Radiographic findings consistent with a coalition in this location include a bridge of bone between the calcaneus and the navicular bone, proximity of the calcaneus to the navicular bone, irregular cortex at the navicular or calcaneal site of the coalition, hypoplasia of the talus, and flattening of the edges of the calcaneus and navicular bone where they abut.

The middle and posterior facets are normally visible on a lateral radiograph, while the anterior facet is obscured as a result of its obliquity and inclination. A possible indication of the presence of a calcaneonavicular bar is the "anteater nose" appearance of the anterior process of the calcaneus. Other secondary signs of coalition seen on lateral radiographs include talar beaking, narrowing of the posterior subtalar joint, rounding of the lateral process of the talus, and failure to observe the middle subtalar joint.

Axial views of the hindfoot (Harris views) can be helpful in the evaluation of a patient with a talocalcaneal coalition. The patient is positioned while standing on the x-ray cassette, bending forward at the ankle about 10°. The x-ray beam is directed down and forward through the heel and subtalar joint. A beam angle of 45° is recommended. Performed correctly, this view projects the posterior and middle talocalcaneal facets. In the normal foot, the middle and the posterior facets are noted to be at different levels, yet parallel. A talocalcaneal bar most commonly occurs in the middle facet, and if the coalition consists of bone, the joint will be obliterated. If the coalition is made of cartilage or fibrous tissue, then the facet will be irregular and angled at its medial border, and the posterior facet will appear horizontal. If the angle of the middle facet is more than 20°, a coalition most likely is present.

In difficult diagnostic cases, a bone scan is considered a good screening test. Increased stress on the joint surfaces next to the coalition usually causes an accumulation of tracer.

Although a calcaneonavicular bar is best seen on the lateral oblique view of the foot, a CT scan is the most reliable test in the evaluation of a talocalcaneal coalition. CT visualizes the anatomy well, helps in surgical planning, quantitates the amount of joint involvement, and can evaluate the joints for degenerative changes. Cortical bridging and/or marrow continuity may be seen with ossified bars. Joint space narrowing, irregularity, abnormal angulation of the joint, and/or enlargement of the sustentaculum tali or the adjacent talus may be seen on CT with fibrous or cartilaginous bars. Talocalcaneal coalitions are best seen on coronal views, and calcaneonavicular coalitions are best seen on long axis or sagittal views.

In skeletally immature individuals, and in those with a possible cartilaginous or fibrous bar, MRI is the best test to order. Continuity of the marrow space (high signal) or cortical bridging (diffuse low signal) may indicate the presence of a tarsal coalition. Cartilaginous bars may show a continuation of the joint cartilage without a normal joint space. Intermediate to low signal material bridging the joint may indicate a fibrous coalition.

Initially, nonsurgical treatment is recommended for calcaneonavicular and talocalcaneal bars. Orthotic devices, such as a UCB orthosis, and shoe modifications, including a medial heel wedge or a Thomas heel, may be helpful. Anti-inflammatory medications also may be helpful. In more severe cases, a short leg walking cast may be used for 4 to 6 weeks. A cast not only decreases inflammation but also allows healing of a fractured or injured bar.

With failure of nonsurgical treatment, and before there are degenerative changes in the hindfoot, excision of the coalition can be performed with good results. Isolated subtalar fusion may be recommended for failed talocalcaneal resections. Failed subtalar fusions and failed excision of calcaneonavicular bars may be treated with triple arthrodesis. Kumar and associates[43] reviewed the surgical treatment of 18 tarsal coalitions. Three feet had resection with no material interposition, 6 had resection with interposition of fat, and 9 had resection with interposition of half of the tendon of the FHL. Eight feet had excellent results, 9 feet had good results, and 1 foot had a poor result due to recurrence of the coalition. Kumar and associates[43] demonstrated that excision of the coalition gives good results, but they did not separate results based on types of coalition or the type of interposition material used. They recommended using half of the FHL as an interposition material because it did not require a second incision and was a simple dissection.

Salomao and associates[44] reviewed 32 tarsal coalitions in 22 children. These patients were treated with resection of the bar and interposition of an autogenous free fat graft. Seventy-eight percent of the patients became pain-free, and 22% reported some residual pain. Sixty-nine percent of the feet had partial correction of the deformity, and 75% had an increase in subtalar motion.

Both of these studies clearly demonstrate that in children, excision of the bar offers relief of symptoms and good function. Although double, triple, or isolated subtalar arthrodesis remains a recognized treatment in older patients, it is possible to excise symptomatic bars in patients who do not demonstrate degenerative changes. The foot is immobilized for around 2 weeks to allow time for the soft tissues to heal and inflammation to decrease. At this time, the patient starts range-of-motion exercises and weightbearing as tolerated.

It should be noted that there have been reports of partial reformation of the bar in 23% to 48% of patients and complete recurrence in up to 10% of patients.[45,46]

In summary, if a tarsal coalition is asymptomatic, no treatment is necessary. If the coalition becomes symptomatic, the conservative treatment described above is tried. If there are no degenerative changes, the bar may be resected. If the foot is in a functional, plantigrade position, it will probably do well after resection of the coalition. If a structural deformity is present, such as varus or inversion of the forefoot, an orthotic device, used to correct these deformities, may be helpful after the excision of the coalition. If degenerative changes are present or resection fails, arthrodesis is recommended. A double arthrodesis, incorporating the subtalar joint and the talonavicular joint is the recommended fusion.

## SINUS TARSI SYNDROME

In the past, sinus tarsi syndrome was described as posttraumatic pain over the sinus tarsi and a feeling of instability in the hindfoot.[47,48] In 1958, O'Connor[47] reported on 45 cases of sinus tarsi syndrome. The diagnosis was based on subjective features including pain over the lateral side of the foot that increased with direct pressure over the sinus tarsi. A feeling of hindfoot instability usually was present. The pain was eliminated with an injection of local anesthetic into the sinus tarsi. Fourteen of the cases that O'Connor reported were cured with excision of the fatty tissue and ligaments in the sinus tarsi.[47]

Most reports of patients with sinus tarsi syndrome have noted a history of at least 1 severe ankle sprain, although other cases were attributed to inflammatory arthritis, gout, pes cavus, pes planus, or chronic subtalar instability. Taillard and associates[48] reported on 21 patients with the following clinical signs: (1) pain over the lateral aspect of the foot that increased with direct pressure over the sinus tarsi and was most severe when standing or walking on uneven surfaces; (2) instability of the hindfoot on uneven ground; (3) feelings of pain and instability relieved with injection of a local anesthetic into the sinus tarsi; (4) no instability of the ankle joint on clinical or radiographic examination; and (5) no abnormalities on routine radiographs of the foot.

Fifteen of Taillard and associates' patients eventually had surgery, which involved a resection of the tissue filling the lateral half of the sinus tarsi. They[48] reported the following results after surgery: 11 excellent, 3 good, and 1 poor.

Frey and associates[36] recently reported on a retrospective review of 21 patients who had subtalar arthroscopy. The patients were evaluated in the following areas: preoperative diagnosis, preoperative tests and clinical evaluation (including MRI and stress tests), intraoperative findings, postoperative diagnosis, complications, and clinical outcome. Although sinus tarsi syndrome was reported as a preoperative diagnosis in 14 patients, in all cases, the diagnosis of sinus tarsi syndrome was changed at the time of arthroscopy. The postoperative diagnoses were 10 interosseous ligament tears, 2 cases of arthrofibrosis, and 2 degenerative joints.

The patients were treated with an arthroscopic debridement of all pathologic tissue, including torn ligaments, scar tissue, inflamed synovium, and any material impinging into the posterior or anterior joints. Using a subjective scale to evaluate postoperative results, there were 9 (43%) excellent, 9 (43%) good, and 3 (14%) poor results.

## INTEROSSEOUS LIGAMENT INJURIES

During inversion sprains to the ankle, the ligaments of the subtalar joint are often injured. The ligaments may be stretched, partially torn, or completely torn. Seventy-four percent (49 patients) of the subtalar arthroscopies performed in my practice between 1988 and 1996 had a diagnosis of interosseous ligament tear confirmed at the time of surgery. Most of these patients suffered an injury to the interosseous ligaments after an inversion injury to the ankle and hindfoot. Twenty-seven of the feet with ligament injuries had hyalinization of the torn ligament ends, with subsequent impingement of the thickened material into the anterior aspect of the posterior subtalar joint. This lesion is referred to as the subtalar impingement lesion (STIL) (Fig. 10).

The diagnosis of interosseous ligament injury and impingement is made primarily on subjective findings: tenderness over the sinus tarsi, feelings of instability in the hindfoot, and pain relief after injection of local anesthetic into the sinus tarsi. These findings are nearly identical to those reported in the past for sinus tarsi syndrome. When the interosseous ligaments are torn, the MRI findings may be consistent with scar, ganglion cyst, or interosseous ligament disruption. The interosseous ligaments are seen best on sagittal and coronal views. Even with considerable experience, the diagnosis of interosseous ligament tear is not an easy one to make on MRI.

The treatment of tears of the interosseous ligaments of the subtalar joint is similar to that of

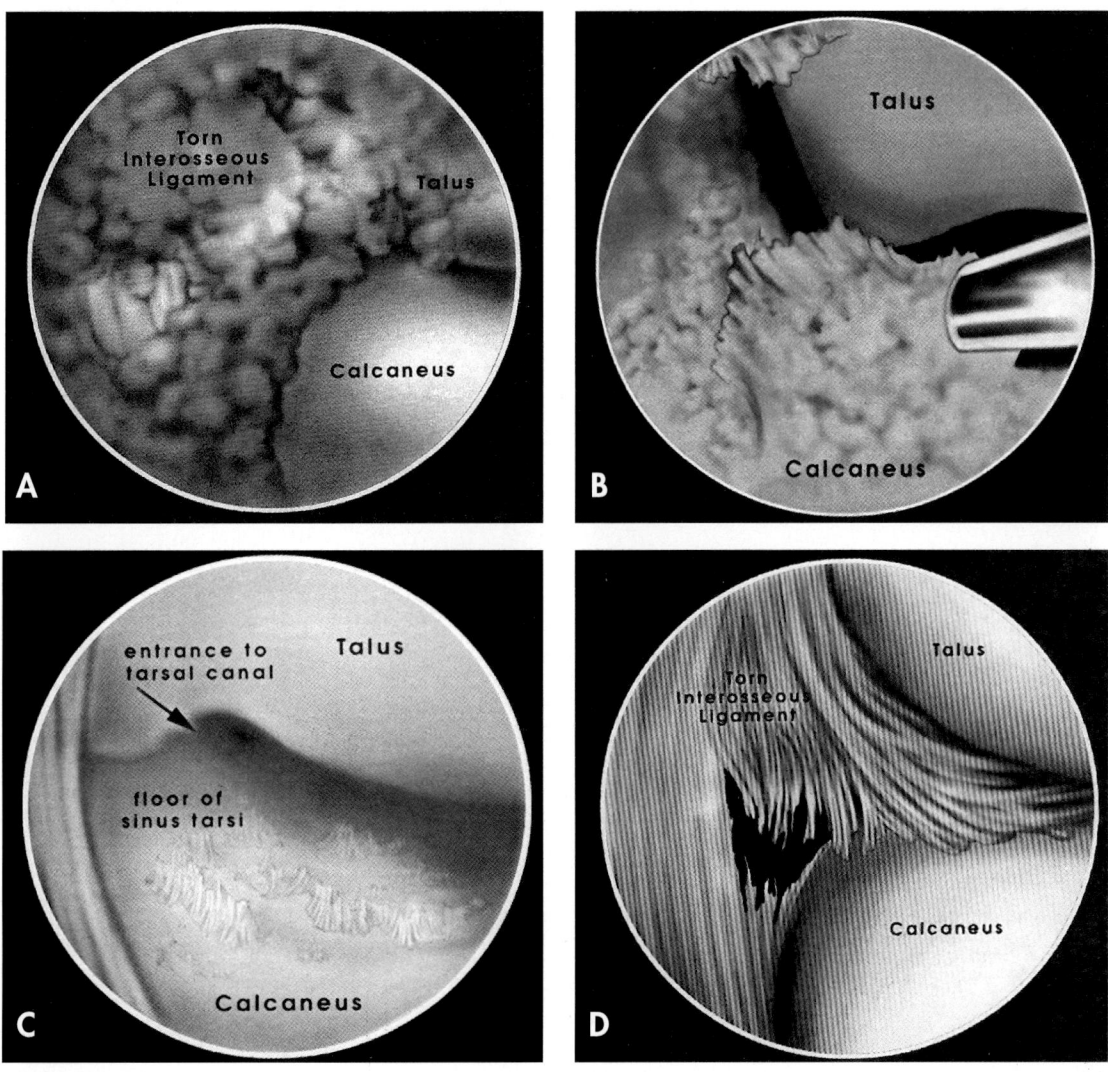

**FIGURE 10**
The subtalar impingement lesion (STIL) is a hyalinization of the torn interosseous ligament. **A,** This material may impinge in the area of the sinus tarsi and the anterior aspect of the posterior subtalar joint. Another case of an interosseous ligament tear before debridement **(B),** during debridement **(C),** and after debridement **(D).**

injury to the lateral collateral ligaments of the ankle. Initial treatment should include anti-inflammatory medication, ice, rest, elevation, and compression. This is followed with range of motion, Achilles tendon stretching, and peroneal strengthening. The final phase of treatment includes proprioception training, conditioning, agility, and a return to sports. An ankle brace with a hindfoot lock may be used for 3 to 6 weeks or until the patient has completely regained range of motion and peroneal strength.

If the patient develops signs and symptoms of instability, this should be treated as directed under subtalar instability. If the patient develops pain and signs of impingement in the subtalar joint, a trial of physical therapy should be ordered, even if the condition is chronic. Anti-inflammatory medications and an ankle brace with a hindfoot lock are recommended. A cortisone injection into the sinus tarsi, angled toward the anterior aspect of the posterior subtalar joint, may be helpful in treating the inflammation and pain and also distinguishing pain in the subtalar joint from that in the lateral gutter of the ankle. If nonsurgical treatment fails, a debridement of the damaged tissue should be undertaken. This can be done as an arthroscopic or open procedure.

## POSTERIOR IMPINGEMENT

Posterior impingement is defined as impingement between the posterior tibial joint surface, the talus, and/or the calcaneus. It can be acute or chronic from trauma and repetitive stress. Posterior impingement is secondary to a plantarflexion injury and can involve any part of the posterior anatomy including the posterior tibia-talus-calcaneus interval.

Because of its location in the posterior ankle joint, a normal os trigonum can become symptomatic in positions of extreme plantarflexion. These positions are not uncommon in ballet and soccer. Once injured, many dancers will attempt to compensate for the loss of ankle plantarflexion by placing the foot in an improper position. The dancer may start to assume a more inverted posture en pointe, a process called "sickling." This position can decrease impingement of the posterior structures but may place increased loads on the anterior talofibular ligament that predispose the dancer to frequent ankle sprains. Calf strain, pain at the plantar aspect of the foot, and curling of the toes are also typical compensatory problems that result from efforts to force the foot into a better en pointe position.

The condition of impingement of the os trigonum is referred to as posterior ankle block, posterior ankle impingement, and the os trigonum syndrome. The condition is initially treated with activity modification, nonsteroidal anti-inflammatory agents, and immobilization. Confirmation of the diagnosis may be made with an injection of local anesthetic agent into the area.

Chronic impingement of the soft tissues, which include the capsule and synovium, can result in a thick inflamed capsule and can result in the development of calcified inflammatory tissue. A prominence of the os calcis can also become impinged on examination. Pain is reproduced by moving the ankle and the foot into extreme plantarflexion. Any of these posterior injuries may be associated with FHL tendinitis.

Posterior impingement and fractures of the ankle may occur at the same time as an ankle sprain. These patients often have a history of having sustained an inversion injury to the ankle. Initial radiographs taken in an emergency room may be read as negative and the diagnosis missed. Typically, a patient demonstrates tenderness on deep palpation anterior to the Achilles tendon but posterior to the talus. Posterior pain may be reproduced by placing the ankle in extreme plantarflexion and may be increased by resisted plantar or dorsiflexion of the great toe. Usually no gross ligament laxity is demonstrated.

Tibial plafond and/or posterior talus changes may be present on careful inspection of radiographs, bone scan, CT, or MRI. Typically, the posterior process of the talus fractures from the main body of the talus and may resemble the os trigonum. A 30° oblique radiograph has been recommended to distinguish fractures of the posterior process from the os trigonum. This fracture is usually larger and extends into the body of the talus.

A bone scan will demonstrate increased uptake in the posterior ankle area when a fracture is present. Other diagnostic studies, which can be helpful, include lateral radiographs in flexion and extension to identify impinging structures (Fig. 11).

Posterior impingement often improves with rest alone. Conservative treatment includes rest, ice, anti-inflammatory medication, avoidance of forced plantarflexion, and casting for 4 to 6 weeks. Physical therapy includes progressive resistive exercises and strengthening. Protective dorsiflexion taping is recommended when the patient returns to sports. If there is an established nonunion, casting is not recommended for initial treatment. Conservative treatment was reported to be successful in about 60% of the patients in 1 series.[23,49] Surgical excision is recommended in the remaining patients, with good results expected. The approach to the posterior ankle for excision of the injured structures is either medial or lateral. When it is necessary to directly observe, protect, or repair the neurovascular structures and the flexor tendons, the medial approach is recommended.[26] The lateral approach gives a more direct approach to the posterolateral processes and os trigonum and is recommended for isolated injuries of these structures. A cast is not required postoperatively. The patient is kept nonweightbearing during the inflammatory phase and begins rehabilitation after 2 weeks. Rehabilitation includes range-of-motion exercises, followed by flexibility, strengthening, and proprioception exercises.

## SUBTALAR ARTHROSCOPY

### INDICATIONS

Indications for subtalar arthroscopy include arthrofibrosis, calcaneonavicular coalition, osteochondral lesions, fractures of the anterior process

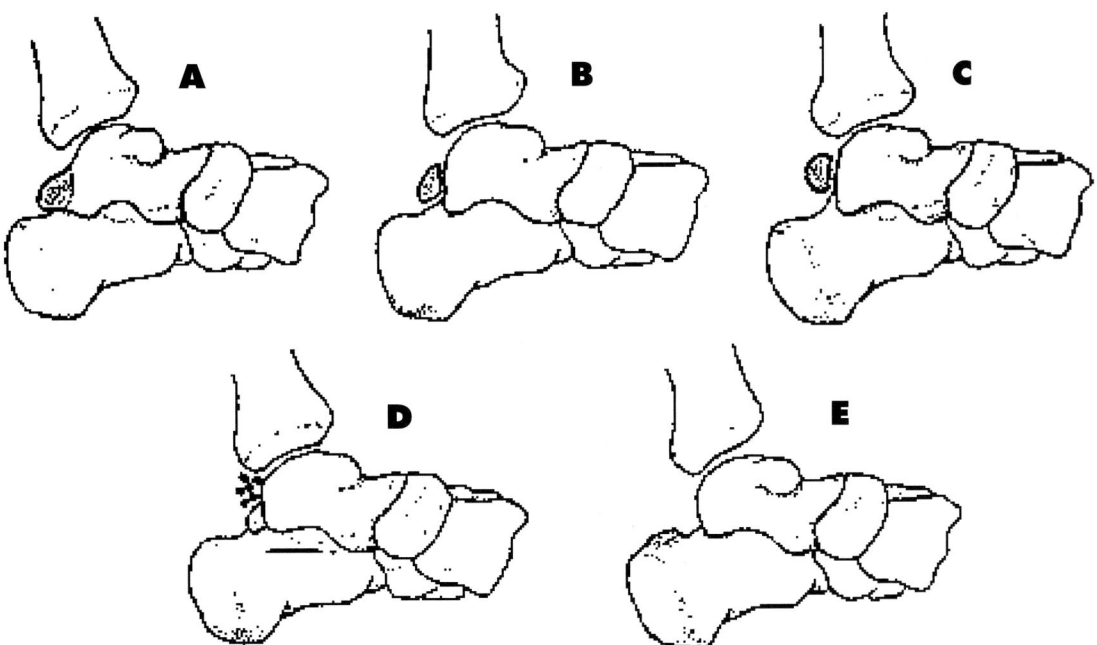

**FIGURE 11**
Anatomic structures involved in posterior ankle impingement including **A**, a large posterior process; **B**, an os trigonum; **C**, a fractured posterior process or separated os trigonum; **D**, calcific inflammatory tissue; or **E**, a prominent posterior process of the os calcis. (Reproduced with permission from Hedrick MR, McBryde AM: Posterior ankle impingement. *Foot Ankle Int* 1994;15:2–8.)

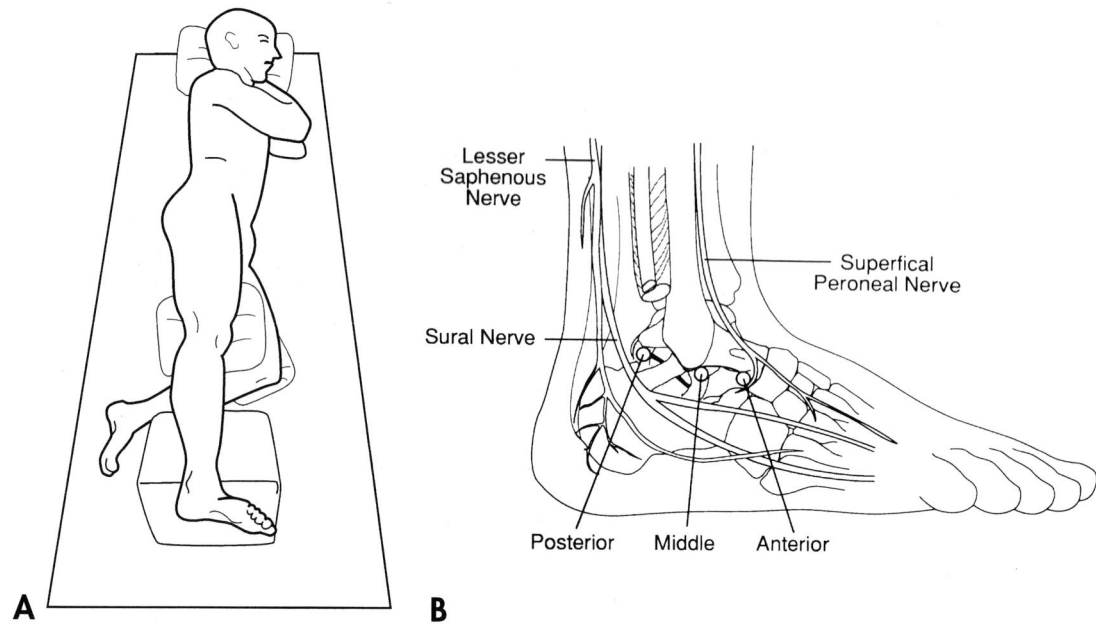

**FIGURE 12**
**A,** Patient is placed in a lateral decubitus position with the extremity to undergo surgery on top. **B,** The location of the anterior, lateral, and middle portals for subtalar joint arthroscopy.

of the calcaneus, fractures of the lateral process of the talus, degenerative joint disease, synovitis, interosseous ligament tears, instability, capsulitis, chronic pain in the sinus tarsi, STIL, arthrodesis of the subtalar joint, and resection of the os trigonum.

## ARTHROSCOPIC TECHNIQUE

The arthroscopic technique follows the initial description of Parisien and Vangsness.[50] They described an anterior and posterior portal. Frey and associates[36,51] noted the importance of adding a third, middle portal. Local, general, spinal, or epidural anesthesia can be used for this procedure. The patient is placed in the lateral decubitus position with the extremity to undergo surgery on top (Fig. 12). Padding should be placed between the lower extremities, as well as under the contralateral extremity to protect the peroneal nerve. The contralateral extremity should be bent to 90° at the knee. A bolster should be placed distally under the upper extremity to suspend the foot and the leg. A thigh tourniquet is recommended for hemostasis. An invasive or noninvasive distracter can be added if necessary for observation but usually is not required.

Three portals are available for observation and instrumentation of the subtalar joint. The anterior portal is placed 2 cm anterior and 1 cm distal to the tip of the lateral malleolus. The middle portal is placed just distal and inferior to the tip of the lateral malleolus. The posterior portal is placed 1 cm proximal to the tip of the fibula and anterior to the Achilles tendon. If the posterior portal is placed too proximal, the posterior ankle joint will inadvertently be entered. If the posterior portal is placed too anterior, the sural nerve and saphenous vein are at risk for injury.

The anterior portal is identified first with an 18-gauge spinal needle, and the joint is inflated with a 50-ml syringe. If the needle is in the joint, backflow will be observed. The needle is removed and a small skin incision is made. The subcutaneous tissue is gently spread using a mosquito clamp. Using the same path, an interchangeable cannula with a semiblunt trocar is placed, followed by the 2.7-mm 30° oblique arthroscope. An arthroscopic pump is recommended, but continued inflation of the joint with a 50-mm syringe is an alternative method to distend the joint until a second portal is established and gravity inflow provided.

The middle portal is now placed under direct observation using an 18-gauge needle and outside-in technique. Once seen, the needle is removed and replaced with an interchangeable cannula. The lateral aspect of the posterior facet and the interosseous ligament are seen well from the anterior portal with instrumentation in the middle portal. If there is synovitis or scar tissue present, the middle portal can be used for debridement. The posterior portal can be placed at this time using the same outside-in technique.

A diagnostic arthroscopic examination is performed, viewing from distal to proximal the posterolateral aspect of the interosseous talocalcaneal ligament, the lateral capsule and its small recess, the articular cartilage of the posterior facets of the talus and calcaneus, and the posterior pouch of the joint with its synovial lining (Fig. 13).

The arthroscope may now be moved to the posterior portal for examination of the interosseous talocalcaneal ligaments, the lateral recess, the reflection of the calcaneofibular ligament, the lateral talocalcaneal ligament, the posterior facet articular cartilage, and the os trigonum and lateral process of the talus.

The middle portal can be used for observation. If the arthroscope is pointed distally, the interos-

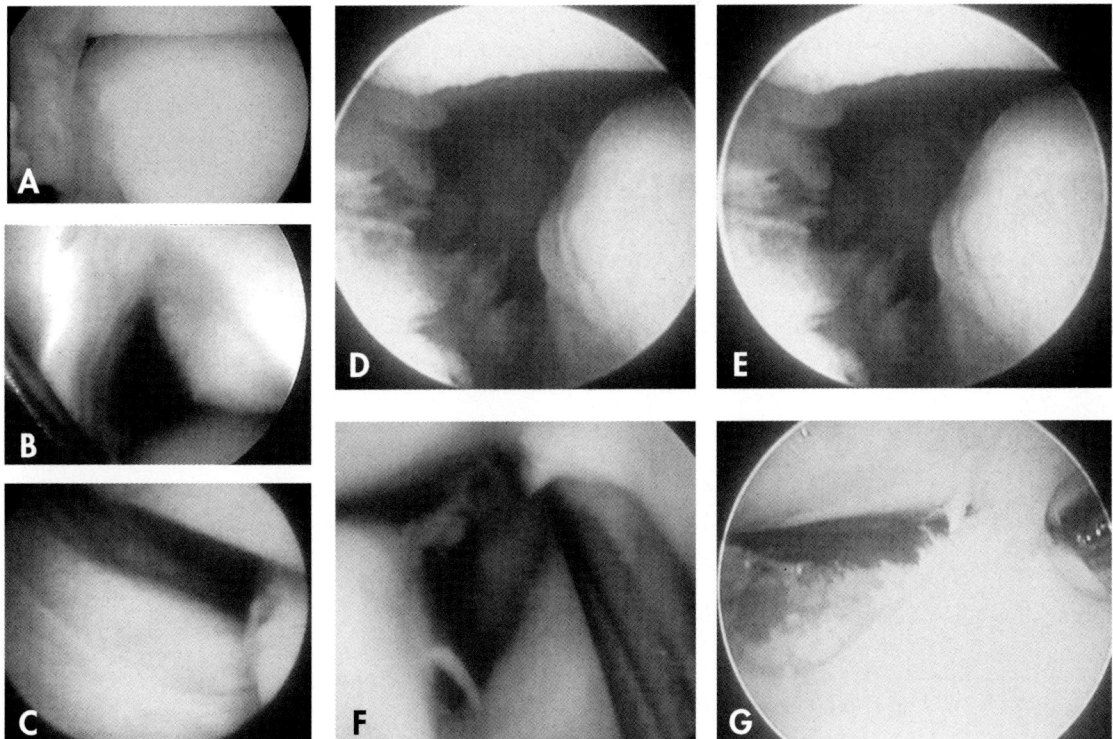

**FIGURE 13**
Arthroscopic anatomy of the subtalar joint. With the arthroscope in the anterior portal of a right foot, **A** shows the lateral capsule and posterior subtalar joint, **B** shows the attachment site on the talus of the lateral talocalcaneal ligament, **C** shows the calcaneal attachment site of the same ligament, **D** shows the posterior lateral pouch of the subtalar joint as the scope is passed from anterior to posterior, and **E** shows the posterior pouch, with Stieda's process and the posterior portal under direct visualization. **F**, The scope remains in the anterior portal and is retracted into the sinus tarsi where the talocalcaneal interosseous ligament is seen. **G**, The scope moves across the floor of the sinus tarsi to the anterior process of the calcaneus. The tip of the shaver is at the origin of the bifurcate ligament.

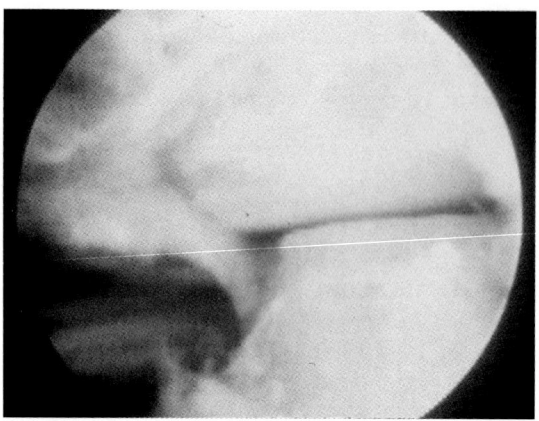

**FIGURE 14**
The anterior and middle facets are seen only if the arthroscope is passed through the interosseous ligaments or there is a significant tear of the ligaments.

seous ligament is seen and if the arthroscope is pointed proximally, the posterior facet is seen.

It is rare to see the anterior and middle facets of the subtalar joint. They can, however, be seen if the interosseous ligament is torn or the arthroscope is passed through the ligament into the anterior compartment of the subtalar joint (Fig. 14).

## POSTOPERATIVE CARE

If the subtalar arthroscopy is performed alone, a bulky dressing is applied and the patient is kept nonweightbearing for 4 to 5 days. On postoperative day 5, the patient begins weightbearing as tolerated and range-of-motion exercises. The sutures are removed on postoperative day 10 to 14 and formal physical therapy is begun with range of motion, progressive resistive exercise, proprioception training, and modalities to decrease inflammation. The patient should be able to return to full activities at 6 to 12 weeks postoperatively.

## RESULTS

Frey and associates[36] reviewed 49 subtalar arthroscopies performed on joints with the following diagnoses: 74% interosseous ligament injuries, 14% arthrofibrosis, 8% degenerative joint disease, and 4% fibrous coalitions of the calcaneonavicular articulation. A subjective scale was designed to evaluate the postoperative results in the above study. Excellent results indicated that there was no pain and no life-style restrictions. Good results indicated that there was improvement but some pain and life-style restrictions. Poor results indicated that the patient had not improved or was worse. With an average follow-up of over 4 years, the following results were observed: 47% excellent results, 47% good results, and 6% poor results. All of the patients with poor results subsequently had a successful subtalar fusion.

There were 5 reported complications, which included 3 cases of neuritis involving branches of the superficial peroneal nerve, 1 case of sinus tract formation, and 1 case of a superficial wound infection that occurred in the patient with the sinus tract formation. The 3 cases of neuritis were treated successfully with cortisone injections and physical therapy. The patient with the sinus tract formation and superficial wound infection was treated successfully with antibiotics, wound care, and subsequent total contact casting.

## REFERENCES

1. Close JR, Inman VT (ed) : *The Action of the Ankle Joint*. Berkeley, CA, University of California, 1952.

2. Wright DG, Desai SM, Henderson WH: Action of the subtalar and ankle-joint complex during the stance phase of walking. *J Bone Joint Surg* 1964;46A:361–382.

3. Karlsson J, Eriksson BI, Renstrom PA: Subtalar ankle instability: A review. *Sports Med* 1997;24:337–346.

4. Brantigan JW, Pedegana LR, Lippert FG: Instability of the subtalar joint: Diagnosis by stress tomography in three cases. *J Bone Joint Surg* 1977;59A:321–324.

5. Clanton TO: Instability of the subtalar joint. *Orthop Clin North Am* 1989;20:583–592.

6. Evans DL: Recurrent instability of the ankle: A method of surgical treatment. *Proc R Soc Med* 1953;46:343–344.

7. Schon LC, Clanton TO, Baxter DE: Reconstruction for subtalar instability: A review. *Foot Ankle* 1991;11:319–325.

8. Cimmino CV: Fracture of the lateral process of the talus. *Am J Roentgenol* 1963;90:1277–1280.

9. Hawkins LG: Fracture of the lateral process of the talus: A review of thirteen cases. *J Bone Joint Surg* 1965;47A:1170–1175.

10. McCrory P, Bladin C: Fractures of the lateral process of the talus: A clinical review. "Snowboarder's ankle". *Clin J Sport Med* 1996; 6:124–128.

11. Mukherjee SK, Pringle RM, Baxter AD: Fracture of the lateral process of the talus: A report of thirteen cases. *J Bone Joint Surg* 1974; 56B:263–273.

12. Backman S, Johnson SR: Torsion of the foot causing fracture of the anterior calcaneal process. *Acta Chir Scand* 1953;105:460–466.

13. Bradford CH, Larsen I: Sprain-fractures of the anterior lip of the os calcis. *N Engl J Med* 1951; 244:970–972.

14. Christopher F: Fracture of the anterior process of the calcaneus. *J Bone Joint Surg* 1931; 13:877–879.

15. Dachtler HW: Fractures of the anterior superior portion of the os calcis due to indirect violence. *Am J Roentgenol* 1931;25:629–631.

16. Degan TJ, Morrey BF, Braun DP: Surgical excision for anterior-process fractures of the calcaneus. *J Bone Joint Surg* 1982;64A:519–524.

17. Gellman M: Fractures of the anterior process of the calcaneus. *J Bone Joint Surg* 1951; 33A:382–386.

18. Green W: Fractures of the anterior-superior beak of the os calcis. *NY St J Med* 1956;56:3515–3517.

19. Jahss MH, Kay BS: An anatomic study of the anterior superior process of the os calcis and its clinical application. *Foot Ankle* 1983;3:268–281.

20. Levine J, Kenin A, Spinner M: Non-union of a fracture of the anterior superior process of the calcaneus: Case report. *J Bone Joint Surg* 1959; 41A:178–180.

21. Piatt AD: Fracture of the promontory of the calcaneus. *Radiology* 1956;67:386–390.

22. Sarrafian SK: Osteology, in Sarrafian SK (ed): *Anatomy of the Foot and Ankle: Descriptive, Topographic, Functional.* Philadelphia, PA, JB Lippincott, 1983, pp 35–106.

23. Shepherd FJ: A hitherto undescribed fracture of the astragalus. *J Anat Physiol* 1882;18:79–81.

24. Paulos LE, Johnson CL, Noyes FR: Posterior compartment fractures of the ankle: A commonly missed athletic injury. *Am J Sports Med* 1983; 11:439–443.

25. Hamilton WG: Stenosing tenosynovitis of the flexor hallucis longus tendon and posterior impingement upon the os trigonum in ballet dancers. *Foot Ankle* 1982;3:74–80.

26. Marotta JJ, Micheli LJ: Os trigonum impingement in dancers. *Am J Sports Med* 1992;20:533–536.

27. Ferkel RD: Subtalar arthroscopy, in Ferkel RD, Whipple TL (eds): *Arthroscopic Surgery: The Foot and the Ankle.* Philadelphia, PA, Lippincott-Raven, 1996, pp 231–254.

28. Brodsky AE, Khalil MA: Talar compression syndrome. *Am J Sports Med* 1986;14:472–476.

29. Burkus JK, Sella EJ, Southwick WO: Occult injuries of the talus diagnosed by bone scan and tomography. *Foot Ankle* 1984;4:316–324.

30. DeLee JC, Curtis R: Subtalar dislocation of the foot. *J Bone Joint Surg* 1982;64A:433–437.

31. Harper MC: The lateral ligamentous support of the subtalar joint. *Foot Ankle* 1991;11:354–358.

32. Pipkin G: The os trigonum. *The Spectator* 1956;1–3.

33. Heilman AE, Braly WG, Bishop JO, Noble PC, Tullos HS: An anatomic study of subtalar instability. *Foot Ankle* 1990;10:224–228.

34. Laurin CA, Ouellet R, St.-Jacques R: Talar and subtalar tilt: An experimental investigation. *Can J Surg* 1968;11:270–279.

35. Kato T: The diagnosis and treatment of instability of the subtalar joint. *J Bone Joint Surg* 1995; 77B:400–406.

36. Frey C, Feder KS, DiGiovanni C: Arthroscopic evaluation of the subtalar joint: Does sinus tarsi syndrome exist? *Foot Ankle Int* 1999;20:185–191.

37. Mann RA: Functional anatomy of the ankle joint ligaments, in Griffin PP (ed): *Instructional Course Lectures XXXVI.* Park Ridge, IL, American Academy of Orthopaedic Surgeons, 1987, pp 161–170.

38. Larsen E: Tendon transfer for lateral ankle and subtalar joint instability. *Acta Orthop Scand* 1988;59:168–172.

39. Chrisman OD, Snook GA: Reconstruction of lateral ligament tears of the ankle: An experimental study and clinical evaluation of seven patients treated by a new modification of the Elmslie procedure. *J Bone Joint Surg* 1969; 51A:904–912.

40. Gould N: Repair of lateral ligament of ankle. *Foot Ankle* 1987;8:55–58.

41. Scranton PE Jr: Treatment of symptomatic talocalcaneal coalition. *J Bone Joint Surg* 1987; 69A:533–539.

42. Harris BJ: Abstract: Anomalous structures in the developing human foot. *Anat Rec* 1955;121:399.

43. Kumar SJ, Guille JT, Lee MS, Couto JC: Osseous and non-osseous coalition of the middle facet of the talocalcaneal joint. *J Bone Joint Surg* 1992; 74A:529–535.

44. Salomao O, Napoli MM, de Carvalho AE Jr, Fernandes TD, Marques J, Hernandez AJ: Talocalcaneal coalition: Diagnosis and surgical management. *Foot Ankle* 1992;13:251–256.

45. Andreasen E: Calcaneo-navicular coalition: Late results of resection. *Acta Orthop Scand* 1968; 39:424–432.

46. Kulik SA Jr, Clanton TO: Tarsal coalition. *Foot Ankle Int* 1996;17:286–296.

47. O'Connor D: Abstract: Sinus tarsi syndrome: A clinical entity. *J Bone Joint Surg* 1958;40A:720.

48. Taillard W, Meyer JM, Garcia J, Blanc Y: The sinus tarsi syndrome. *Int Orthop* 1981;5:117–130.

49. Hedrick MR, McBryde AM: Posterior ankle impingement. *Foot Ankle Int* 1994;15:2–8.

50. Parisien JS, Vangsness T: Arthroscopy of the subtalar joint: An experimental approach. *Arthroscopy* 1985;1:53–57.

51. Frey C, Gasser S, Feder K: Arthroscopy of the subtalar joint. *Foot Ankle Int* 1994;15:424–428.

# ARTHROSCOPIC TREATMENT OF OSTEOCHONDRAL LESIONS, SOFT-TISSUE IMPINGEMENT, AND LOOSE BODIES

RICHARD D. FERKEL, MD

## OSTEOCHONDRAL LESIONS OF THE TALUS

Osteochondral lesions of the talus (OLT) represent a difficult diagnostic and therapeutic problem to the surgeon treating the athlete. The purpose of this section is to describe what is known about these lesions and to identify appropriate methods of diagnosis and treatment to facilitate the patient's return to athletic competition.

## TERMINOLOGY

A variety of terms have been used to describe these lesions, including transcondylar fractures, osteochondral fractures, osteochondritis dissecans, talar dome fractures, and flake fractures. This problem in terminology has arisen, in part, from the lack of a clearly defined and universally accepted etiology. The term "osteochondritis dissecans" literally translated suggests separation or an inflammatory lesion of the cartilage and bone; however, because this term has very little relevance to the actual pathophysiology of the condition, the more general term OLT is recommended.

## HISTORY

In 1856, Alexander Munro[1] was the first to describe osteochondral loose bodies of the ankle joint and implicated trauma as the cause. König[2] coined the term "osteochondritis dissecans" when he noted loose bodies in other joints such as the knee, which he thought were due to spontaneous osteonecrosis. Barth,[3] in 1898, described the same lesion, but thought it was due to an intra-articular fracture. However, he was not sure whether the etiology was trauma or whether these lesions could arise spontaneously. In 1922, Kappis[4] first applied the term "osteochondritis dissecans" to the ankle joint. This term generally was used until 1959, when Berndt and Harty[5] wrote their classic treatise, in which they theorized that the lesion had a traumatic etiology and coined the term "transchondral fracture of the talus."

## ETIOLOGY

The etiology of OLT remains controversial. In 1966, Campbell and Ranawat[6] concluded that osteochondritis is a disease process resulting in pathologic fracture through necrotic bone as a result of ischemia. This argument is supported by the fact that trauma is not documented in all cases of OLT. In addition, some argue that a history of an ankle injury may not be a statistically significant etiologic factor because eliciting such a history is not uncommon. Moreover, this lesion has also been associated in the literature with alcohol abuse, steroids, emboli, and hereditary and endocrine factors.

Other evidence to support nontraumatic causation for OLT is that some families have multiple affected members with these lesions. In addition, patients who have simultaneous involvement of the ankle and other joints have been reported occasionally. Furthermore, 10% of patients have lesions in both ankles.

Trauma, however, remains most popular as the etiology for OLT. The trauma theory suggests that the lesion represents the chronic phase of a compressed or avulsed talar dome fracture. A distinct episode of macrotrauma or repetitive microtrauma resulting from overuse may contribute to initiation of the lesion in a person with a predisposition to talar dome ischemia. An osteonecrotic process will result in a subchondral fracture, and collapse may exist. Progression and symptomatology may result in alteration of joint biomechanics, with increased joint pressures resulting in the forcing of synovial fluid into the fracture site, preventing healing. Because the subchondral fracture has no soft-tissue attachment and no blood or nerve supply, it is highly susceptible to osteonecrosis.

The trauma theory was initially introduced by Berndt and Harty,[5] who analyzed their own patients and also subjected 15 cadaveric ankle specimens to a variety of forces. More recent studies have also supported a traumatic etiology. Canale and Belding[7] reported on their patients with talar dome lesions and found 100% of the lateral lesions and 64% of the medial lesions were associated with trauma. They analyzed their data, compared them with data from studies by Yvars,[8] Röden and associates,[9] and Marks,[10] and theorized that the medial lesions were either traumatic or nontraumatic and the lateral lesions were usually traumatic in origin. In addition, Flick and Gould[11] reviewed reports of OLT in over 500 patients. They found that 98% of the lateral talar dome lesions and 70% of the medial talar dome lesions were associated with a history of trauma.[11] Other authors [12–17] have also found a high percentage of the lesions (75% or greater) to be associated with trauma (Fig. 1).

## INCIDENCE

OLTs are relatively uncommon. However, their exact incidence is probably underestimated because many patients with these lesions are asymptomatic and plain radiographs may miss the diagnosis in a significant number of cases. Incidence of OLT has been reported as ranging from 0.09% of all talar fractures, based on a

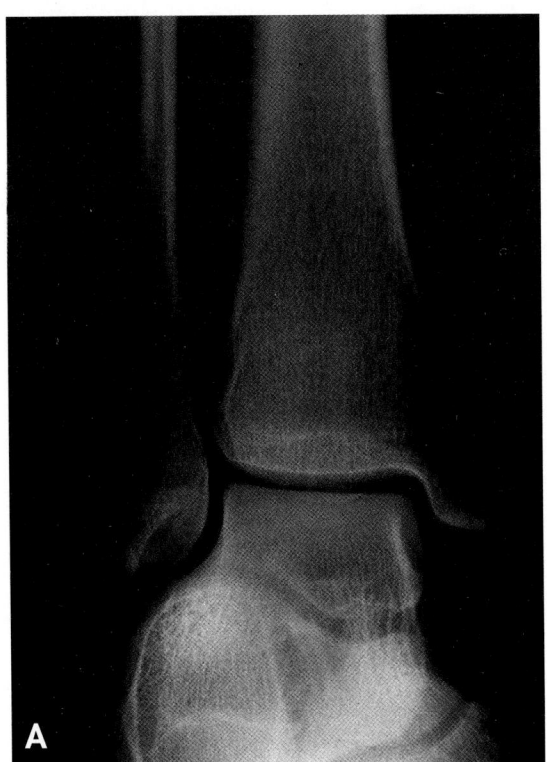 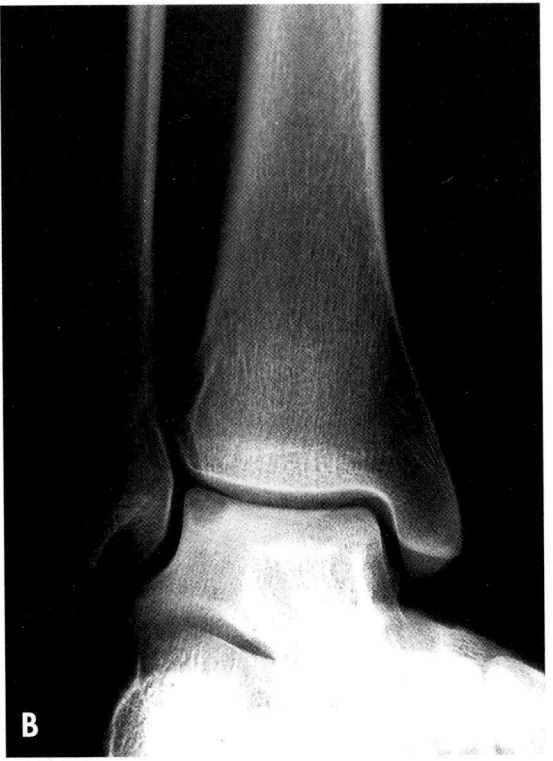

**FIGURE 1**
Development of osteochondral lesions of the talus (OLT). **A,** Mortise radiograph of right ankle without evidence of OLT. **B,** Mortise radiograph 3 years later, after traumatic episode, demonstrating large osteochondral lesion of the anterolateral talus.

series reported during World War II, to 6.5% of 133 sprains studied by Bosien and associates.[18] Ankle lesions appear to represent 4% of all cases of osteochondritis dissecans reported in the literature.[19] Several series indicate the incidence of bilateral lesions ranges around 10%.[5,20] The average age of most patients with OLT is between 20 and 30 years, with males slightly more predominant.

## LOCATION

Osteochondral lesions on the medial aspect of the talar dome occur in the middle or posterior third; whereas lateral lesions occur primarily in the anterior or middle portion. However, there are exceptions; lesions in the anteromedial corner and posterolateral corner and central lesions also are seen, and on some occasions these lesions may occur in multiple sites. In most series, medial OLT lesions are more common than lateral ones. Medial lesions are usually deeper and cup-shaped and are not displaced, whereas lateral lesions are usually shallow or wafer-shaped and often are displaced and elevated by the levering effect of the distal tibia.

## MECHANISM OF INJURY

The mechanism of injury for OLT differs, depending on whether the lesion is medial, lateral, or central. In addition, more than one mechanism can be associated with similar appearing lesions. Berndt and Harty[5] used cadavers to reproduce the mechanisms of medial and lateral lesions. Lateral talar lesions were replicated by a strong inversion force to a dorsiflexed foot with the tibia internally rotated. Medial talar lesions were reproduced by a strong inversion force to a plantarflexed foot with external rotation of the tibia on the talus. Berndt and Harty[5] theorized that the principal force causing both medial and lateral talar dome lesions was torsional impaction. With lateral lesions, as the foot is dorsiflexed and strongly inverted, the lateral talar margin is impacted and compressed against the medial articular surface of the fibula, causing a shearing and compressing component that could potentially displace the osteochondral fragment.

In contrast, medial talar dome lesions are reproduced when the foot is inverted and plantarflexed with the tibia in external rotation, causing the posteromedial edge of the talar dome to impact against the posteromedial tip of the tibia, leading to increased shear stress.

The shear stress that is the inversion stress on the ankle joint creates a moment of force that can be resolved along coordinate axes. A fracture may occur along the line of the shear force component. Whether the medial or lateral aspect of the dome is involved may depend on whether the ankle is in a dorsiflexed or plantarflexed position. The amount of the fragment that may be displaced depends on whether the shear stress is greater than the ultimate strength of the bone or cartilage. If the ultimate shear stress is greater than the strength of the bone, articular cartilage may deform momentarily but will remain intact while the underlying bone fractures. However, if the magnitude of the resultant shear stress is greater than the ultimate strength of both articular cartilage and bone, a complete lesion is produced and the fragment may be displaced from its bed.[21]

Yao and Weis[22] believed that lateral lesions were caused by eversion of the foot with the ankle dorsiflexed and the tibia internally rotated on the talus. Furthermore, they hypothesized that medial lesions were produced by inversion of the foot with the ankle plantarflexed.

Because many lesions, particularly on the medial side of the talar dome, occur without known trauma, no single mechanism can explain each case. Particularly in the group where no specific history of injury or associated etiologic factor can be documented, idiopathic osteonecrosis or repetitive microtrauma may be postulated.

## CLINICAL PRESENTATION

Although some patients seek help immediately after an acute ankle injury, most seek help after chronic ankle pain does not resolve with conservative treatment. Usually an inversion injury of the lateral ligamentous complex is described as the mechanism of injury, but in some cases no injury is recalled. Symptoms usually are intermittent and can include stiffness; pain of a deep, aching nature aggravated by weightbearing; swelling; catching; clicking; locking; and less commonly, giving way.

Physical examination is often nonspecific or vague. Patients may have tenderness either medially or laterally, pain with range of motion, limited range of motion, swelling, weakness, or evidence of instability. Patients with posteromedial osteochondral lesions have more pain anteriorly with the ankle plantarflexed and posteriorly with the ankle dorsiflexed. Lateral lesions elicit pain with direct pressure or with forced plantarflexion. Different studies suggest that the average duration of symptoms before definitive diagnosis is made ranges from 4 months to 2 years.

## RADIOLOGIC EVALUATION

After a careful examination, 3 views of the ankle should be obtained: anteroposterior (AP), mortise, and lateral. Although the diagnosis of OLT has traditionally been made using plain radiographs, many plain radiographs do not demonstrate the lesion. Alexander and Barrack[23] reported that mortise and AP views can be taken in various degrees of plantarflexion and dorsiflexion to show the lesion.

In patients with persistent pain, a bone scan is a useful, inexpensive way to screen for OLT. If positive, further investigation using other types of studies is indicated.

In 1988, Zinman and associates[24,25] reported on 32 patients with OLT and found computed tomography (CT) scans to be superior to plain radiographs for both diagnosis and follow-up. CT scans can be done with or without contrast, and should always be done in two planes, both the axial (transverse) and coronal. Bilateral hindfoot CT scans are helpful to assess both hindfeet at the same time and to determine if bilateral lesions are present. Contrast may assist in evaluating the articular surface, either pre- or postoperatively, and in determining healing.

Magnetic resonance imaging (MRI) has been advocated as being preferable to CT in evaluating OLT lesions. Anderson and associates[17] compared CT with MRI in 24 cases and found that CT scans failed to detect stage I lesions in four patients, while MRI clearly showed these lesions. Ferkel and associates[26] reviewed radiographs, CT, MRI, and intraoperative videos of 80 patients, and concluded that CT in the coronal and axial planes is the study of choice when there is a known diagnosis of OLT. However, if radiographs and clinical examinations are not diagnostic, then MRI may be more valuable because of its ability to image both bone and soft tissue and assess articular cartilage. Generally, CT is preferable to MRI when trying to understand the cortical outlines of the lesion and exact size, because in some cases MRI, with imaging of surrounding edema of the lesion, may indicate the lesion to be bigger than what is found at the time of surgery.

## CLASSIFICATION AND STAGING

Berndt and Harty's classification[5] was based primarily on plain radiographs of acute ankle injury. However, because the lesion is often chronic and not always well seen on plain radiographs, the usefulness of this classification is limited. In 1980, Ferkel and associates[27] developed a CT staging system that corresponds to the stages described by Berndt and Harty, but accounts for the extent of osteonecrosis, subchondral cyst formation, and the separation of fragments that are not seen radiographically. In 1995, this system was further verified by Ferkel and associates;[26] in both studies, all preoperative CT scans of over 100 patients were viewed in a double-blinded manner. In this four-stage classification, CT scans were evaluated in both the coronal and axial (transverse) planes (Fig. 2, Table 1).

MRI has also been used to stage osteochondral lesions of the talus.[28,29] Anderson and associates[17] compared CT, bone scan, and MRI results in 24 patients with a history of ankle injury. Group 1 had ankle symptoms but normal radiographs, whereas group 2 were symptomatic but had abnormal radiographs. They found bone scans useful in diagnosing lesions in patients who had normal radiographs. In addition, in most cases results obtained using CT were comparable to those obtained with MRI; however, CT

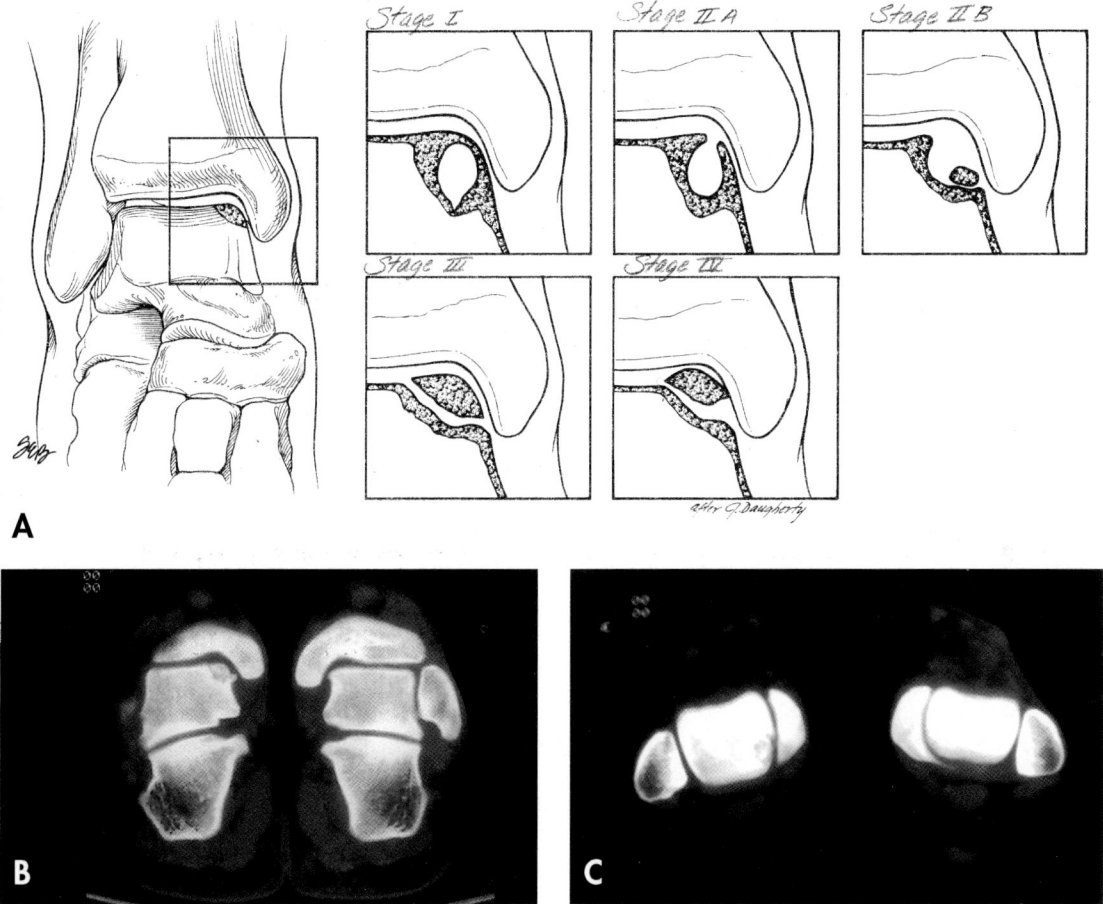

**FIGURE 2**
**A,** Drawings based on computed tomography (CT) scans demonstrating stages I through IV of the classification developed by Ferkel and Sgaglione.[27] (Adapted with permission from Ferkel RD: *Arthroscopic Surgery: The Foot and Ankle.* Philadelphia, PA, Lippincott-Raven, 1996. Susan Brust, medical illustrator.) **B,** Coronal CT scan demonstrating a stage III osteochondral lesion of the right ankle. **C,** Axial CT scan demonstrating a posteromedial osteochondral lesion, stage III, of the right ankle.

did not indicate the diagnosis in four patients with stage I MRI lesions. Based on this study, they developed an MRI classification[17] (Table 2).

De Smet and associates[30] compared MRI and arthroscopy of 14 patients. They believed that MRI was an accurate predictor of fragment stability in their case group.

In 1995 Ferkel and associates[26] reviewed preoperative radiographs, CT or MRI scans, and intraoperative videotapes of 80 patients. Results were correlated with the previously mentioned MRI and CT staging systems also were correlated with a new arthroscopic staging system (Table 3). The results showed that CT is the test of choice if there is a known diagnosis of OLT. However, if radiographic and clinical findings are not diagnostic, then MRI is more valuable because of its ability to image both soft tissue and bone. In addition, no significant correlation was found between CT and MRI scans and the arthroscopic appearance of the lesions, except with stage III and stage IV problems. In this study, arthroscopic appearance

## TABLE 1
### COMPUTED TOMOGRAPHY CLASSIFICATION

| Stage | Description |
| --- | --- |
| Stage I | Cystic lesion within dome of talus, intact roof on all views |
| Stage IIA | Cystic lesion with communication to talar dome surface |
| Stage IIB | Open articular surface lesion with overlying nondisplaced fragment |
| Stage III | Undisplaced lesion with lucency |
| Stage IV | Displaced fragment |

(Reproduced with permission from Ferkel RD, Sgaglione NA: Arthroscopic treatment of osteochondral lesions of the talus: long term results. *Orthop Trans* 1993;17:1011.)

## TABLE 2
### MAGNETIC RESONANCE IMAGING (MRI) CLASSIFICATION

| Stage | Description |
| --- | --- |
| Stage I | Subchondral trabecular compression |
| | Plain radiograph normal, positive bone scan |
| | Marrow edema on MRI |
| Stage IIA | Formation of subchondral cyst |
| Stage II | Incomplete separation of fragment |
| Stage III | Unattached, undisplaced fragment with presence of synovial fluid around fragment |
| Stage IV | Displaced fragment |

(Reproduced with permission from Anderson IF, Crichton KJ, Grattan-Smith T, Cooper RA, Brazier D: Osteochondral fractures of the dome

## TABLE 3
### SURGICAL GRADE BASED ON ARTICULAR CARTILAGE

| Grade | Description |
| --- | --- |
| Grade A | Smooth, intact but soft or ballottable |
| Grade B | Rough surface |
| Grade C | Fibrillations and fissures |
| Grade D | Flap present or bone exposed |
| Grade E | Loose, undisplaced fragment |
| Grade F | Displaced fragment |

(Reproduced with permission from Ferkel RD, Cheng MS, Applegate GR: Abstract: A new method of radiologic and arthroscopic staging for osteochondral lesions of the talus. Proceedings of the American Academy of Orthopaedic Surgeons 62nd Annual Meeting, Orlando, FL. Rosemont, IL, American Academy of Orthopaedic Surgeons,

the lesion. They graded the arthroscopic appearance of the lesion as grade I, intact, firm shiny cartilage; grade II, intact with soft cartilage; and grade III, free of cartilage. Pritsch and associates[12] believed that the arthroscopic appearance of the OLT was the most important determinant for treatment because it was more accurate than plain radiographs.

## TREATMENT INDICATIONS

Controversy exists as to the appropriate treatment for OLT. Some of the confusion is a result of the uncertainty about the etiology and nature of the lesion. Limitations of current imaging systems also contribute. In addition, there is no long-term study of the natural history of untreated OLT because patients rarely are seen for this problem unless they are symptomatic. Seven of 11 patients in a series reported by Lindholm and associates[31] were asymptomatic when treated conservatively with an average follow-up of 7 years. Reports of other studies suggest that the lesion may show radiographic failure to heal over a long period of follow-up, but this is not incompatible with a successful outcome (asymptomatic ankle). Berndt and Harty[5] and subsequently Canale and Belding[7] concurred that stage I and II lesions, whether medial or lateral, should be treated nonsurgically.

correlated better with eventual results than did CT and MRI.

Pritsch and associates[12] examined the radiographs and performed arthroscopy on 24 patients. They found that an increase in radiographic stage of the lesion did not necessarily predict increasing fragmentation or loosening of

They also suggested nonsurgical treatment initially for stage III medial lesions, and surgical treatment only if symptoms persisted. Surgical treatment was recommended for stage III lateral lesions and all stage IV lesions, based on the Berndt and Harty classification. Although there were only 29 patients with 31 osteochondral lesions in the Canale and Belding study, it is frequently cited to justify surgical treatment of stage III and IV osteochondral lesions.[7]

Other authors have argued that surgical treatment is superior to conservative care. Blom and Strijk[20] suggested that it was sometimes difficult to distinguish stage II from stage III Berndt and Harty lesions and advocated surgical treatment. Yvars,[8] Alexander and Lichtman,[32] O'Farrell and Costello,[33] and Flick and Gould[11] also advocated surgical treatment. Alexander and Lichtman[32] and Flick and Gould[11] agreed that a delay in surgical treatment resulting from a trial of nonsurgical therapy did not adversely affect the later surgical results. However, the latter authors, in a review of 22 patients with 2-year follow-up also argued that surgical treatment yielded better results than conservative therapy, even with a number of stage II lesions.

Pettine and Morrey[15] also recommended a period of immobilization for OLT and even suggested nondisplaced medial stage III lesions had a chance of healing with conservative treatment. They believed that a delay in diagnosis had an adverse effect on outcome, but delaying surgery for less than 1 year did not.

### My Indications

In MRI scan stage I and II lesions, conservative treatment is advocated initially in both acute and chronic situations. This should include 6 to 12 weeks of immobilization by brace or cast, with the length determined by the size of the lesion, chronicity of the lesion, patient age, and healing potential. Currently, there is no good evidence that nonweightbearing in a cast is any better than weightbearing, nor is the duration of nonsurgical treatment clear from previously published studies. At this time, protected weightbearing is allowed. If the patient remains symptomatic after the proposed conservative program, then surgical treatment is advocated.

Surgical treatment is advocated for all symptomatic CT and MRI stage III and IV lesions. The only exception to this rule is children with stage III lesions whose growth plates have not closed at the distal tibial and fibular epiphyses. For these patients, initial conservative treatment with casting or immobilization before surgical intervention is recommended.

### Beware

It is critical to operate on OLT only in symptomatic cases. This axiom appears obvious, but some situations can be misleading. For example, a 19-year-old male college basketball player twisted his left ankle and had exquisite pain along the anteromedial and posteromedial aspects of the talus and medial malleolus. MRI showed bilateral OLT, but with significant bone bruising of the medial malleolus on the injured side without bone edema at the OLT site (Fig. 3). In this case,

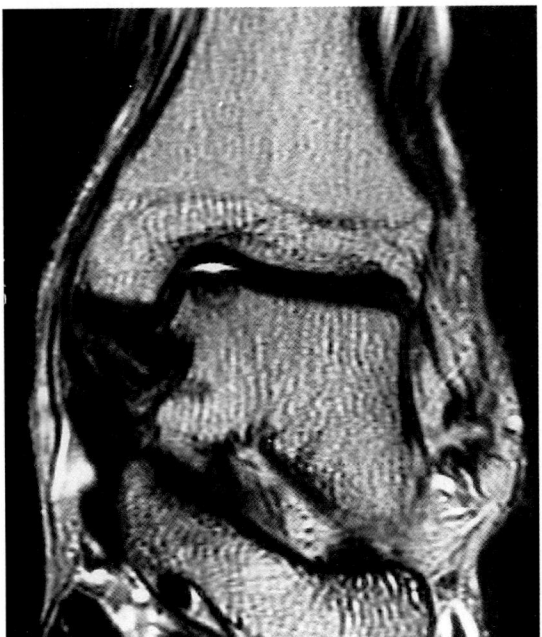

**FIGURE 3**
Coronal T2-weighted magnetic resonance image of the left ankle demonstrating an osteochondral lesion without evidence of bony edema. Other views demonstrated a contusion of the medial malleolus.

conservative treatment and enough patience allowed the patient's symptoms to resolve. He then returned to play for his college season without incident. It is vital that the surgeon always proves that the OLT is the source of the pain before performing any surgery for this problem.

## SURGICAL TREATMENT

Surgical treatment of OLT has traditionally involved extensive ankle arthrotomy for excision of loose bodies, joint debridement, and drilling or abrasion at the lesion site. The results of open treatment have been described in numerous studies.[5,7,32-35] Furthermore, a number of methods have been reported for the treatment of posterior lesions, particularly those involving the posteromedial aspect of the talar dome. These include extensive arthrotomy,[19] distal tibial articular surface grooving,[11,36] medial or lateral malleolar osteotomy,[5,7,11,15,32,33,37-39] and percutaneous fluoroscopic drilling.[40] Unfortunately, these approaches require significant tissue trauma and may be associated with nonunion or malunion of the malleoli, postoperative joint stiffness, prolonged rehabilitation, suboptimal cosmetic appearance, and inadequate posterior visualization of the talar dome lesions.

With the development of improved small joint instrumentation, 2.7-mm (30° and 70°) and 1.9-mm (30°) small joint arthroscopes and distraction techniques, ankle arthroscopy has evolved to become a useful tool for both the diagnosis and treatment of OLT[41,42] (Fig. 4). It provides an alternative approach to open procedures, and it also can provide superior visualization of the entire joint surface and improved access to the lesion without an extensive surgical approach. This technique can help to reduce the morbidity associated with ankle arthrotomy or malleolar osteotomy, as well as permit the procedure to be done on an outpatient basis with quicker rehabilitation and functional return.

### Surgical Choices

Controversy exists as to the optimal method to treat full-thickness loss of articular cartilage, such as an OLT. Penetration of the subchondral bone

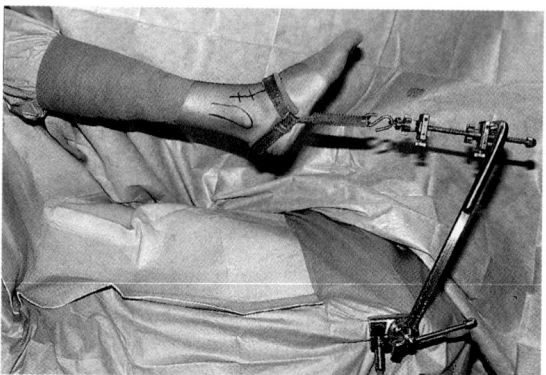

**FIGURE 4**
Noninvasive distraction setup on a right ankle with distraction strap positioned appropriately to allow for anterior and posterior access.

disrupts subchondral blood vessels.[43-45] Subsequently, a fibrin clot forms and fibrocartilaginous repair tissue often forms over the surface to protect it from excessive loading.[38,46] Experimental studies suggest that cells responsible for a new fibrocartilaginous articular surface may enter the fibrin clot from the marrow.[45,47] These cells start as undifferentiated mesenchymal cells and then differentiate into chondroblasts and chondrocytes.

A variety of techniques have been advocated for penetrating subchondral bone to perform cartilage repair, including resecting sclerotic subchondral bone, drilling through subchondral bone,[43,45] abrading the articular surface,[46,48] and creating small-diameter defects (microfractures) with a sharp instrument.[49] Presently, no study has proved the efficacy of one method over another. Recent comparisons of abrasion with drilling for treatment of experimental chondral defects in the rabbit demonstrate that the long-term results of drilling appear to be better than those of abrasion.[50,51]

### Technique

The surgical technique used to treat OLT is the same as has been discussed previously, including the use of small joint instrumentation, 2.7-mm 30° and 70° arthroscopes, and use of anteromedial, anterolateral, and posterolateral portals, as well as accessory portals when necessary. A complete 21-point examination is initially performed, so that not only the talus but the entire tibial articular surface is inspected because it is not uncommon to have associated pathology in patients with these lesions.

### Acute OLT

The principles of treating acute OLT are different than those for chronic lesions. With an acute OLT, the first priority is to carefully identify the lesion via imaging techniques. If the acute lesion is displaced, arthroscopy should be done immediately, and the consent should read "arthroscopy with possible open pinning or removal of osteochondral lesion of the talus." In these acute situations, the lesion should be palpated carefully with a small joint probe, and a decision should be made whether enough bone is attached to the chondral fragment to allow healing if it is reattached. Chondral lesions are generally excised with subsequent debridement of the base. Because the lesion is acute, generally there is good vascularity in the OLT bed; only occasionally is drilling, abrasion, or microfracture necessary.

If enough bone is attached to the loose chondral fragment and the articular cartilage appears healthy, the piece should be reattached. The displaced fragment is reduced with a probe or grasper gently holding the edge to replace the fragment anatomically so it can be temporarily attached with a Kirschner wire (K-wire). Firm fixation is then facilitated with absorbable pins or screws, K-wires, or fibrin glue (Fig. 5).

### Chronic OLT

Before the treatment of chronic OLT, it is critical to identify the lesion correctly with imaging techniques. The lesion is then carefully palpated with a small joint probe through multiple portals, and the decision is made whether the lesion is loose or unstable. Lesions that are not loose can be drilled by transmalleolar or transtalar methods, using 0.045- or 0.062 K-wires. Loose osteochondral lesions should be excised with a banana knife, ring curette, or shaver to healthy bone. The osteochondral talar bed is then treated with drilling, abrasion, or microfracture. Medial lesions are usually central to posterior and require drilling by the transmalleolar or transtalar approach using a small joint drill guide (MicroVector™, Smith and Nephew Endoscopy, Andover, Massachusetts) (Fig. 6). It has been my experience that loose chronic OLT lesions generally do not heal with internal fixation because of a fibrous membrane that separates the lesion from the remaining talar bed. This fibrous mem-

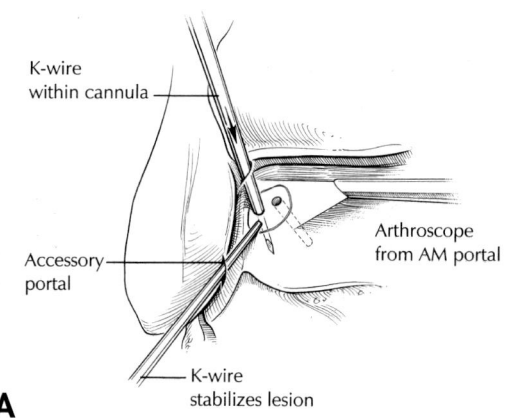
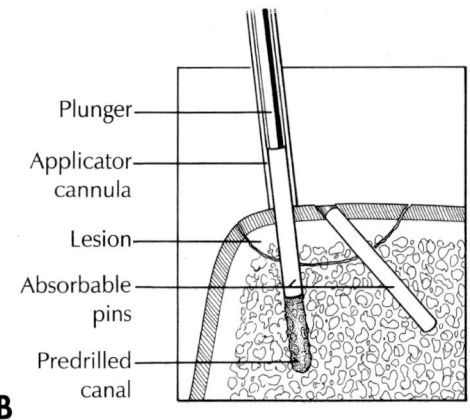

**FIGURE 5**
Acute osteochondral lesion of the talus. **A,** The acute lesion is stabilized so that absorbable pins can be inserted. **B,** Absorbable pins are inserted arthroscopically using a plunger after measuring the appropriate length of the pin and predrilling the hole. AM = anteromedial. (Reproduced with permission from Ferkel RD, Whipple TL (eds): *Arthroscopic Surgery: The Foot and Ankle*. Philadelphia, PA, Lippincott-Raven, 1996; Susan Brust, medical illustrator.)

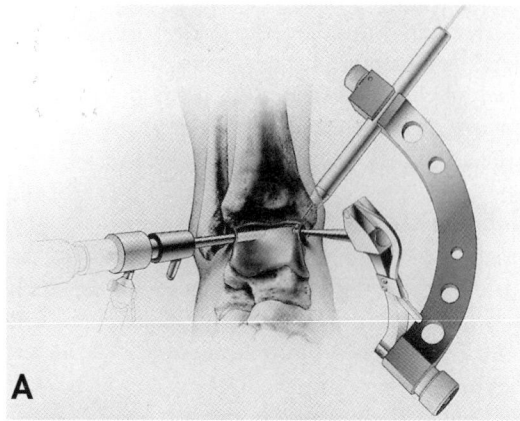
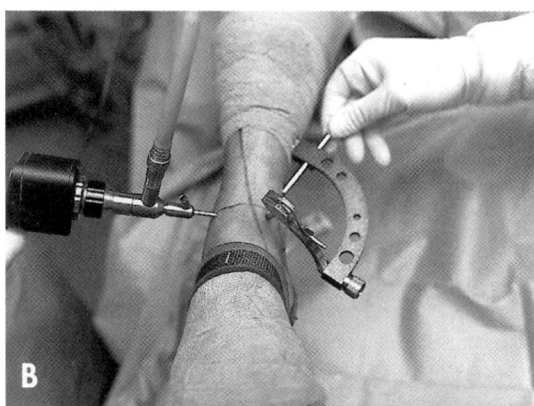
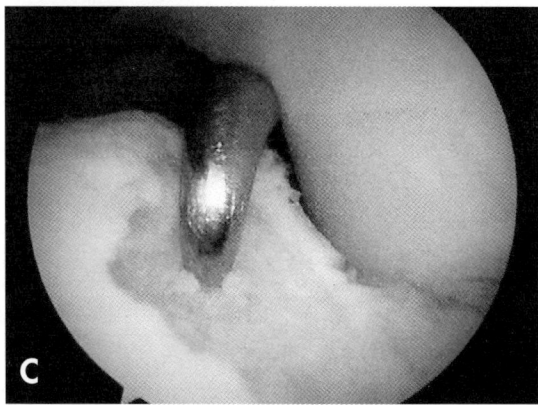

**FIGURE 6**
Chronic osteochondral lesion of the medial talus. **A,** Drawing demonstrating arthroscope in the anterolateral portal and MicroVector™ in the medial portal to facilitate transmalleolar drilling of the osteochondral lesion of the talus. (Copyright © 1995, Richard D. Ferkel, MD) **B,** Intraoperative picture demonstrating setup with distraction strap. **C,** Arthroscopic view from the posterolateral portal, showing introduction and use of the microfracture pick through the anteromedial portal.

brane always needs to be removed to allow bleeding and new formation of fibrocartilage.

The posteromedial osteochondral lesion can be drilled in 4 ways. First, the MicroVector can be used to perform transmalleolar drilling. A small incision is made over the medial malleolus, and the drill guide is inserted through the anteromedial portal while looking through the posterolateral portal. Usually, 0.062 K-wires are used, and the surgeon must be careful to insert the pin into the talar lesion at the correct angle. Once the first pin is inserted, a second method is to use an offset guide to place multiple holes into the talar lesion; alternatively, the drill guide can be reinserted in a different position. Drilling is usually performed at 3- to 5-mm intervals to a depth of 10 mm to potentiate vascular access. A third method is to drill transmalleolarly and dorsiflex and plantarflex the ankle with the pin tip barely exposed from the distal tibia. This allows fewer drill holes through the medial malleolus while gaining extra holes into the talus through each guide pin inserted. It is critical once the pin is drilled into the talus that the ankle not be moved until the pin is removed from across the joint. Otherwise, the pin can bend or break.

The fourth method of drilling is transtalar drilling. This involves using a drill guide to insert a K-wire percutaneously near the sinus tarsi at the junction of the talar neck and body. If the articular surface has been removed, the drill can be extended into the joint surface. However, if a cystic lesion is involved, the tip of the drill is placed just beneath the articular surface, the hole is cored out, and bone graft is inserted from the distal tibia or calcaneus and impacted through a cannula with a plunger into the cystic lesion.

Cystic lesions (CT scan stage I) can be treated by transtalar or transmalleolar drilling, or by bone grafting through a transtalar or medial talar window approach. However, these techniques will work only if the articular surface overlying the cystic lesion is healthy and stable. In CT scan stage IIA lesions, the articular surface has an opening, and the articular cartilage is loose. Frequently the underlying bone will appear hard and sclerotic after the chondral fragment is removed. However, if a true cyst exists, a ring curette or microfracture awl should be used to pop into the cyst area and then excise the entire cyst and fibrous membrane. Often the cyst cavity will be large and deep, and bone grafting should be considered. Using a special arthroscopic cannula system, the bone graft is taken from the calcaneus or distal tibia and inserted into the talar bed.

## TREATMENT OF SPECIFIC LESIONS

### Anterolateral Lesions

Anterolateral or central lesions of the talar dome are best approached through the anteromedial and anterolateral portals. Generally, observation through the anteromedial portal allows instrumentation through the anterolateral portal and inflow through the posterolateral portal. In the acute situation, the fragment can be reduced and pinned through the anterolateral portal. The more common chronic lesion is excised through the anterolateral portal, and drilling, microfracture, or abrasion is performed through this portal as well. Occasionally, the MicroVector can be inserted through the anterolateral portal, and drilling can be done through the fibula or medial malleolus for lesions that are more central and posterior.

### Anteromedial Lesions

These lesions are uncommon and may be treated through the anteromedial portal with observation through the anterolateral portal.

### Posterolateral Lesions

Posterolateral lesions are less common and more difficult to diagnose and treat. After accurate localization, the lesion is carefully evaluated through all 3 portals. Usually these lesions are treated by observing from the anteromedial portal and operating through the posterolateral portal. A 70°-arthroscope can facilitate observation. Occasionally, the lesion is so posterior that the posterior and accessory posterolateral portals are used for observation and treatment. Bone grafting of these lesions is usually done through the posterolateral portal as well.

### Posteromedial Lesions

These lesions are the most common type seen in a chronic situation, and usually occur in the middle or posteromedial dome of the talus. Rarely does a posterocentral lesion occur. It is particularly important in these lesions to make sure the anteromedial portal is established as close to the anterior tibial tendon as possible to allow a straight line of access from anterior to posterior. Otherwise, the surgeon will butt the instruments against the medial malleolus, prohibiting effective instrumentation and treatment.

Most posteromedial lesions are seen through the posterolateral portal, and a banana knife, ring curette, shaver, and burr are used through the anteromedial portal. Transmalleolar drilling is also done through the anteromedial portal or through a transtalar approach, drilling out through the

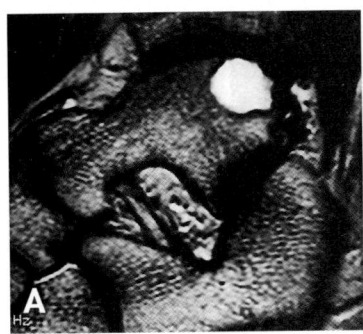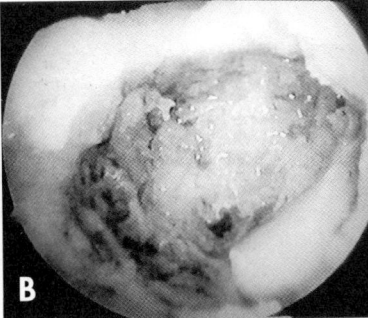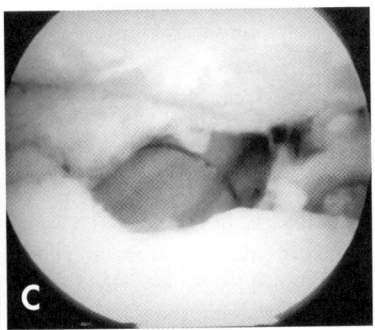

**FIGURE 7**
Posterior talar cyst. **A,** Sagittal T2-weighted magnetic resonance image demonstrating large posterior subchondral cyst. **B,** Arthroscopic picture after cyst cavity has been debrided and curetted. **C,** Insertion of bone graft through posterolateral portal via a cannula system.

sinus tarsi. Bone grafting is done through the posterolateral or anteromedial portals, depending on the size and location of the lesion and the flexibility of the joint to allow extreme dorsiflex or plantarflexion. Cartilage margins should be excised at 90° to the articular surface so as not to undermine or bevel the margins. This "quarry effect" may assist with better clot retention in the defect and subsequent metaplasia to fibrocartilage, with the potential for reconstitution of the articular surface.[21]

### Preferred Technique
All acute displaced OLT are attached with absorbable pins or screws. Patients are immobilized for approximately 2 weeks until the fragment is stabilized, and then gentle active range of motion is encouraged. Patients are kept nonweightbearing for 4 to 6 weeks, depending on the size of the lesion.

Chronic painful stage III and IV lesions are excised and the fibrous membrane removed. A combination of microfracture and transmalleolar or transtalar drilling is performed in the exposed bony bed. Exact treatment is determined by the location and size of the lesion and the density of the bone. Large cystic areas are bone grafted using grafts from the distal tibia or calcaneus. These grafts are obtained using a special graft harvesting system that allows measurement of the exact diameter of the graft and then insertion through an arthroscopic cannula with a plunger and impactor (Fig. 7). The patient is immobilized 1 week, and then early range of motion is initiated. Nonweightbearing varies from 4 to 6 weeks, depending on the size and location of the lesion.

## POSTOPERATIVE CARE
After drilling, abrasion, or microfracture, the tourniquet is deflated and fluid flow is stopped with the suction on. This allows the surgeon to see the area of pathology and to determine whether adequate vascular access has been created over the site. Postoperatively, the wounds are closed with permanent suture and a compression dressing, and a posterior splint is applied with the ankle at 90°. At 1 week, the stitches are removed and a removable posterior splint is made so the patient can initiate range-of-motion exercises four to six times a day while continuing nonweightbearing. Debate still exists as to the appropriate length of time the patient should be nonweightbearing after surgery. Both immediate weightbearing and delay of weightbearing for 2 to 12 weeks are advocated.

After the wounds are healed, formal physical therapy usually is started. Rehabilitation is initiated in the pool, with gentle mobilization and isometric exercises. This is followed by the development of proprioceptive training and further strengthening. Joint loading activities and impact exercise are avoided for at least 3 months and, in some cases, longer, depending on the size and location of the lesion. A four-phase rehabilitation program is used, with the final phase emphasizing return to sports activity. This involves a plyometric exercise program and advanced proprioceptive training.

## RESULTS
Open versus arthroscopic results are summarized in Tables 4 and 5. Arthroscopic results appear to be as good as or better than the open results. My colleagues and I recently reviewed our long-term results to determine current patient function and satisfaction. Between January 1984 and June 1995, 136 consecutive patients have been treated arthroscopically for OLT at the Southern California Orthopedic Institute (SCOI). Sixty-four of these patients fulfilled the criteria, which consisted of a chronic OLT (more than 2 months), treatment by one surgeon, no previous ankle surgery, and no other associated pathology of the ankle joint. The average age of the patients was 32 years, and average length of follow-up was 71 months. Overall, 72% had excellent or good results when the American Orthopaedic Foot and Ankle Society (AOFAS) Hindfoot Score was used for the entire group. We found no correlation between plain radiographs, CT, or MRI staging and clinical results using any of the rating systems, but found good correlation between arthroscopic staging and results (Ferkel RD, Zanotti RM, Komenda GA, personal communication).

**TABLE 4**

**COMPARISON OF ARTHROTOMY TREATMENT RESULTS**

| Study | Year | Cases | Follow-up (Mos) | Average Age (Yr) | Trauma (%) | Good Results (%) |
|---|---|---|---|---|---|---|
| Berndt & Harty[5] | 1959 | 56 | — | 35 | 90 | 79 |
| Mukherjee & Young[37] | 1973 | 10 | 17 | 28 | 100 | 90 |
| Alexander & Lichtman[32] | 1980 | 25 | 65 | 22 | 92 | 88 |
| Naumetz & Schweigel[38] | 1980 | 31 | — | 24 | 84 | 63 |
| Canale & Belding[7] | 1980 | 15 | 134 | 23 | 83 | 73 |
| O'Farrell & Costello[33] | 1982 | 24 | 47 | 24 | 92 | 63 |
| Flick & Gould[11] | 1985 | 19 | 24 | 28 | 91 | 79 |
| Pettine & Morrey[15] | 1987 | 30 | 90 | 12-66 | 85 | 33 |
| Zinman & Reis[25] | 1988 | 28 | 62 | 14-60 | 21 | 82 |

**TABLE 5**

**COMPARISON OF ARTHROSCOPIC TREATMENT RESULTS**

| Study | Year | Cases | Follow-up (Mos) | Average Age (Yr) | Trauma (%) | Good Results (%) |
|---|---|---|---|---|---|---|
| Baker et al[14] | 1986 | 10 | 12.5 | 29 | 100 | 90 |
| Pritsch et al[12] | 1986 | 24 | 30 | 28 | 75 | 75 |
| Parisien[13] | 1986 | 10 / 8 | 24 / 6.5 | 14-40 | 89 | 88 |
| Van Buecken et al[16] | 1989 | 15 | 26 | 23 | 93 | 87 |
| Frank et al[87] | 1989 | 9 | 10-24 | 24 | 66 | 89 |
| Loomer* | 1993 | 19 | 19 | 31 | — | 74 |
| Chin et al[88] | 1996 | 25 | 24 | | 80 | 75 |
| Baker & Morales[89] | 1999 | 12 | 20 | 25 | 75 | 83 |
| Kelberine & Frank[90] | 1999 | 48 | 60 | 26 | — | 75 |
| Kumai et al[86] | 1998 | 18 | 54 | 28 | 56 | 72 |
| Ferkel et al† | 1999 | 50 | 71 | 32 | 73 | 72 |

\* Loomer RL, Personal communication, January 1995.
† Ferkel RD, Zanotti RM, Komenda GA, unpublished data.

## FUTURE TRENDS

Recently, clinical management of articular cartilage defects and degeneration has generated significant research interest in the orthopaedic community. Techniques for treatment of articular cartilage defects that have recently been advocated include marrow and stem cell techniques, periosteal-perichondral grafts, chondrocyte transplantation, and osteochondral autograft and allograft transplantation.[52-54]

Chondrocyte transplantation has been studied extensively in Sweden and is currently undergoing clinical trials in the United States.[55-57] Most patients studied thus far have been treated for lesions of the knee, and very few ankle OLTs have been treated with this technique.[58]

Currently, the most popular new technique for treating OLT is with autogenous osteochondral grafts, and is termed "mosaicplasty." These grafts are taken from a donor site on the supracondylar ridge of the femur and inserted into the osteochondral lesion of the talus by an arthrotomy. A preliminary report indicated excellent results in 11 patients when this technique was used.[59]

With the extensive research now occurring, the problem of healing and regeneration of articular cartilage may have a solution in the future. However, further research is needed to determine the effectiveness of these newer techniques before they can be advocated.

# OSTEOCHONDRAL LESIONS OF THE TIBIA

## ETIOLOGY

Osteochondral lesions of the distal tibia are rare and receive little attention in the orthopaedic literature. The exact etiology of these lesions is unknown. Trauma appears to be the primary etiologic factor, although secondary etiologies are numerous and include abnormal vasculature, embolic events, spontaneous necrosis, hormonal factors, endocrine disorders, and abnormal stress due to malalignment. As has been shown in OLT, lesions in the tibial plafond can cause abnormal stress patterns and can lead to accelerated cartilage wear. This abnormal stress pattern can lead to cancellous bone remodeling and eventual cyst formation.[60]

## SIGNS AND SYMPTOMS

Osteochondral lesions of the distal tibia can present in a nonspecific manner. Patients complain of various chronic symptoms, including pain, stiffness, swelling, locking, and occasionally, instability. On physical examination, pain can be poorly localized to the medial, central, or lateral aspects of the ankle. Possible loss of motion and catching or locking can occur occasionally.

## DIAGNOSTIC EVALUATION

Plain radiographs usually are not helpful in establishing the diagnosis in most cases. Radiographs demonstrate sclerosis around the loosened lesion that is contiguous with the articular surface of the distal tibia. CT scan will help demonstrate the cystic lesion more clearly, as well as determine its exact size and location. MRI also is helpful in the diagnosis; it can demonstrate bone edema and cystic fluid and can help in determining if the overlying cartilage is intact (Fig. 8, *A*).

## TREATMENT

The treatment of osteochondral lesions of the distal tibia is similar to that recommended for treating talar lesions. The ankle is evaluated thoroughly through a 21-point arthroscopic examination using the three-portal technique.[61] Usually, the overlying articular cartilage and the distal tibial cyst are significantly softened and loose. The lesion is debrided with a shaver and curetted with ring and cup curettes down to bleeding bone. If the underlying bone is sclerotic, it can be abraded with a burr (Fig. 8, *B*). Drilling or microfracture of the subchondral bone allows for vascular ingrowth and stimulation of fibrocartilage formation, similar to lesions of the talus.

In some cases where large cystic cavities have formed, it may be helpful to use the MicroVector drill guide to insert a guide pin into the center of the lesion. The cyst is then reamed from a small incision over the medial malleolus, and the resulting hole is bone grafted from the iliac crest, distal tibia, or calcaneus. It is important during bone grafting to observe the lesion arthroscopically and to use an instrument to allow compaction of the bone graft while keeping the graft out of the joint.

Postoperatively, the patients are placed in a posterior splint for 1 week and then the stitches are removed. A compression dressing and remov-

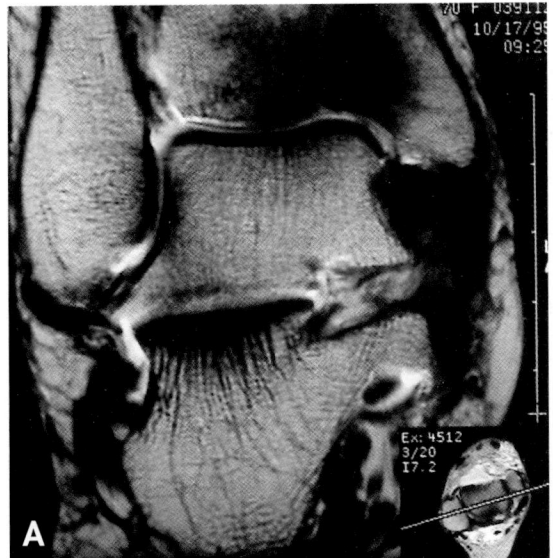 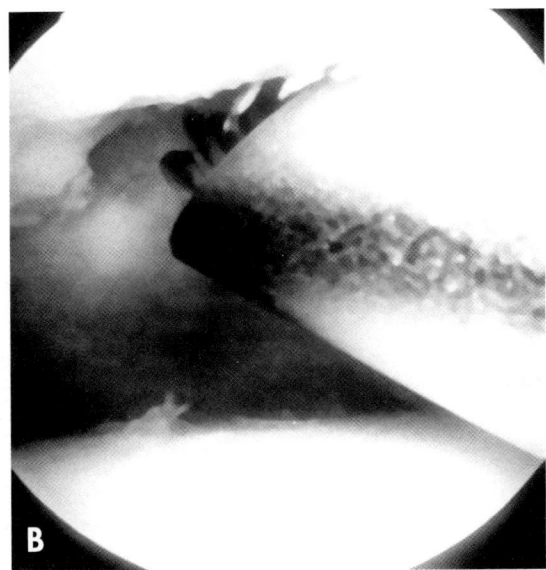

**FIGURE 8**
Osteochondral lesion of the tibia. **A,** Coronal magnetic resonance image with intraarticular gadolinium showing osteochondral lesion of the tibial plateau with chondral irregularity. **B,** Arthroscopic picture showing burring of the osteochondral lesion of the tibia.

able posterior splint are then applied, and active ankle motion is encouraged four times a day while the patient remains nonweightbearing for 4 to 6 weeks. Plain radiographs or CT scans can assist in monitoring the incorporation of the graft into the cystic cavity.

## RESULTS

Few articles discuss osteochondral lesions and results of treatment. Recently, Mologne and Ferkel (unpublished data) studied the first series of 17 patients with osteochondral lesions of the distal tibia. The average age of the patients was 38 years, and a traumatic event was reported by 65% of the patients. The average time from onset of symptoms to surgery was 22 months. Plain radiographs revealed an irregularity or abnormality in only 35%, whereas MRI revealed the lesion in 100% of cases. The average AOFAS Ankle-Hindfoot Score was 55. Eleven patients were found to have isolated osteochondral lesions of the distal tibia (group I), and six patients were found to have osteochondral lesions of both the tibia and talus (group II).

Treatment was as described above.

The average follow-up was 44 months, and the average postoperative AOFAS Ankle-Hindfoot Score was 85. This score averaged 92 for group I and 73 for group II. Using the Modified Weber Score, 82 patients had good and excellent results, with 6% fair and 12% poor (Mologne TS, Ferkel RD, unpublished data).

## SOFT-TISSUE IMPINGEMENT

Ankle sprains are one of the most common injuries in sports. One inversion ankle sprain occurs per 10,000 persons per day.[62–64] At West Point, 30% of cadets suffer an ankle sprain in their 4 years at the school.[65] Most commonly, these involve basketball (45%), volleyball (25%), and soccer (31%). After an ankle sprain, 20% to 40% of patients have some chronic pain.[65–69]

Ankle sprains can occur by a variety of mechanisms. However, the most common injuries are associated with plantarflexion and inversion, or dorsiflexion and inversion. With an inversion injury, the following sequence occurs: torn anterior talofibular ligament, torn calcaneofibular ligament, and torn posterior talofibular ligament. During this sequence, the syndesmotic ligaments anteriorly and/or posteriorly can also be injured. Differential diagnosis of patients with chronic postsprain pain includes OLT, calcific ossicles or loose bodies, peroneal tears or subluxation, tarsal coalition, bone bruises,[70] occult fractures of the talus or calcaneus, degenerative joint disease, nerve entrapment, subtalar dysfunction, reflex sympathetic dystrophy, and soft-tissue impingement. One of the most common causes of chronic pain after an ankle sprain is soft-tissue impingement. This can be seen along the syndesmosis, anterior gutter, syndesmotic interval between the tibia and fibula, or posteriorly in the syndesmosis and posterior gutter.

## ANTEROLATERAL IMPINGEMENT

Because of the mechanism of most ankle sprains, anterolateral soft-tissue impingement of the ankle is commonly seen. Wolin and associates,[71] in 1950, described nine patients with persistent pain and swelling over the anterolateral aspect of the ankle chronically after an inversion sprain. Arthrotomy of the ankle in these patients revealed a massive hyalinized connective tissue extending into the joint from the anteroinferior portion of the talofibular ligament. They called this a "meniscoid" lesion because it looked like a torn meniscus in the knee and believed that repeated tension (or impingement) of this tissue led to pain and swelling in the ankle. Excision of this tissue relieved the patient's symptoms in all cases. A proposed sequence for development of chronic anterolateral soft-tissue impingement is described in Figure 9.

In 1982, Waller[72] described "anterolateral corner compression syndrome." The pain in this syndrome was along the anteroinferior border of the fibula and anterolateral talus and was believed to result from repetitive inversion injuries.

### Anatomy

Soft-tissue impingement is usually located anterolaterally and rarely anteromedially. The borders of

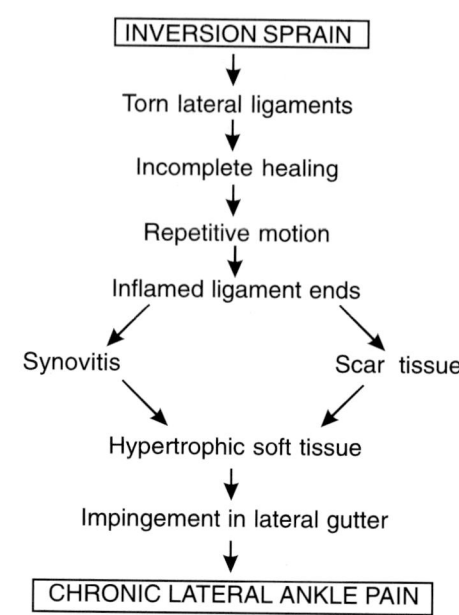

**FIGURE 9**
Sequence of lateral ankle pain.

the lateral gutter of the ankle include the talus medially, fibula laterally, and tibia superiorly, bordered by the anteroinferior tibiofibular ligament (AITF). The anteroinferior section of the lateral gutter is bordered by the anterior talofibular, calcaneofibular, and anterior talocalcaneal ligaments. The posterior and inferior borders are composed of the posterior talofibular, calcaneofibular, and posterior talocalcaneal ligaments (Fig. 10).

Anterolateral soft-tissue impingement of the ankle occurs at three primary sites: (1) the superior portion of the AITF ligament; (2) the distal portion of the AITF ligament, which may involve a separate fascicle; and (3) along the anterior talofibular ligament (ATFL) and lateral gutter near the area of the lateral talar dome (Fig. 10).

### Clinical Presentation

Chronic lateral ankle pain is much more common than chronic medial ankle pain after a sprain. Typically the athlete will complain of persistent, vague anterolateral pain, usually along the anterolateral aspect of the ankle, sometimes involving the syndesmosis and sinus tarsi regions.

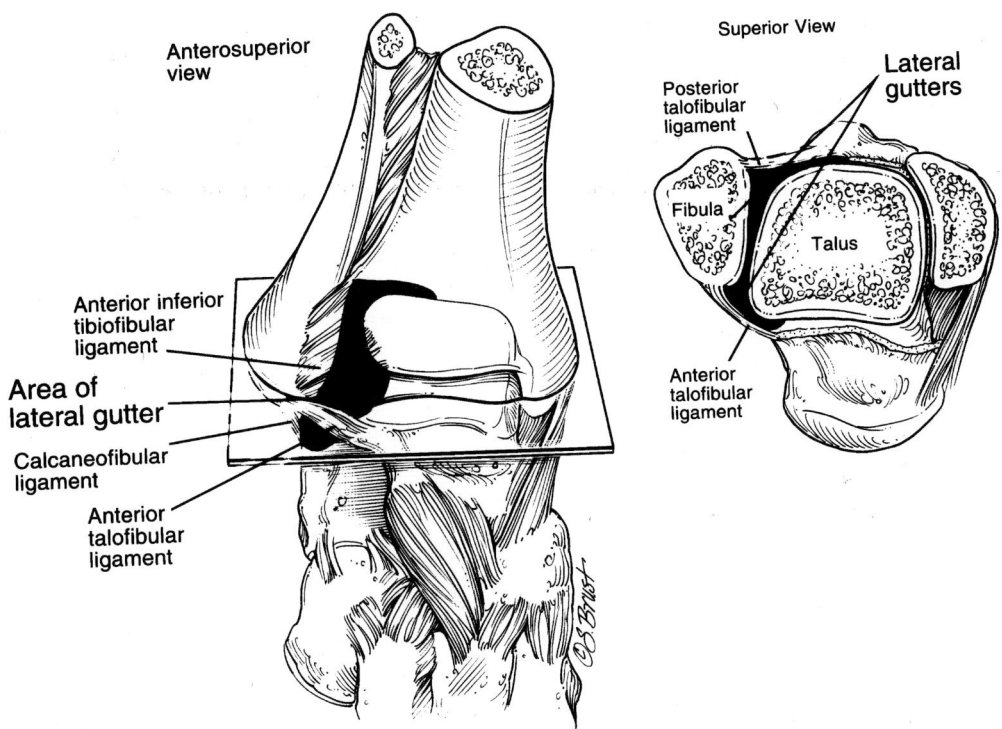

**FIGURE 10**
Lateral gutter anatomy. On the left, the confines of the anterolateral gutter are demonstrated; on the right, axial cross-section showing the extension of the anterior gutter through the articulation of the fibula and the talus to the posterior gutter. (Copyright © 1995, Richard D. Ferkel, MD)

Pain is usually absent at rest and present with most activities, including cutting and pivoting movements. Often the patient has seen several physicians and is frustrated by lack of progress in alleviation of the symptoms. Generally, these patients do not complain of buckling, giving way, or signs of instability.

Physical examination reveals tenderness along the ATFL and lateral gutter, and sometimes along the syndesmosis and calcaneofibular ligament. In addition, pain is frequently noted along the posterior subtalar joint or sinus tarsi, and it is important to differentiate the exact site of pain by careful palpation along the ankle and subtalar region.

Radiologic evaluation may show ossicles along the tip of the fibula and irregularity along the lateral talar dome, consistent with injuries of the ATFL. In some cases, heterotopic bone will be seen in the interosseous space or along the distal portion of the AITF. In most instances, the radiographs are normal, as are CT and MRI scans. MRI may be helpful in diagnosis of anterolateral soft-tissue impingement, possibly showing fluid in the lateral gutter with a torn remnant of the syndesmosis or ATFL. Synovial thickening may also be shown with a low signal-density mass in the anterolateral gutter on the sagittal T1-weighted image (Fig. 11).

### Treatment

Initial treatment should be conservative and include nonsteroidal anti-inflammatories, physical therapy, bracing, orthotics, and steroid injections. Xylocaine injections are also helpful to differentiate pain in the ankle from pain in the subtalar joint.

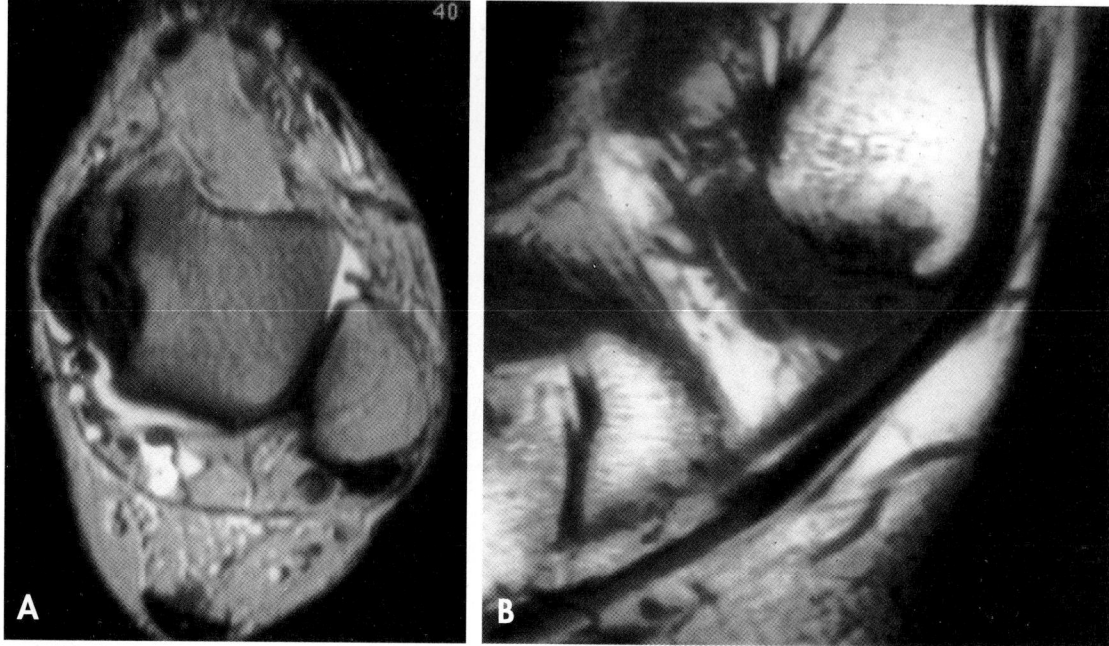

**FIGURE 11**
Magnetic resonance image (MRI) of soft-tissue impingement. **A,** Axial T2-weighted MRI showing fluid in the lateral gutter with torn remnant of the anterior talofibular ligament. **B,** Sagittal T1-weighted MRI showing low signal intensity consistent with anterolateral soft-tissue impingement of the ankle.

When conservative treatment fails, arthroscopic surgery is indicated to alleviate the patient's symptoms. At arthroscopy, positioning can be done using either the supine, lateral decubitus, or 90° flexed position. To see the entire ankle, 2.7-mm or 4.0-mm 30° and 70° arthroscopes are used. Motorized shavers, burrs, graspers, and baskets are used to treat the associated pathology, and soft-tissue distraction is used to see the entire joint and facilitate inflow as well as treatment.

### Preferred Method

The patient is placed in the supine position with a nonsterile thigh holder, and the foot is prepared and draped. All anatomic landmarks are carefully marked out and the ankle is distended with 10 ml of saline from the anteromedial portal. A 2.7-mm short 30° video arthroscope with a 2.9-mm interchangeable cannula is inserted. The anterolateral portal is made carefully under direct vision to permit good access to the anterolateral gutter, while inflow is done through the posterolateral portal.

During the procedure, the soft-tissue distraction force should be varied because too much distraction can occlude the anterolateral compartment of the ankle, making observation more difficult. Dorsiflexion of the ankle relaxes the anterior capsule and opens up the lateral gutter. The entire ankle is inspected using a 21-point examination,[61] and the sites of pathology are noted. Arthroscopy usually reveals synovitis surrounding the AITF, both in front and behind, as well as synovitis in the ATFL. Fibrosis and scar bands of the lateral gutter and chondromalacia of the talus and fibula are also seen in some instances (Fig. 12, *A* to *C*). In some instances, a small ossicle or loose body may be hidden in the soft tissues at the tip of the fibula, and, rarely, thick adhesive scar bands may be noted extending from the anterolateral aspect of the distal tibia to the lateral gutter (ie, meniscoid bands).

Treatment usually involves using the 70° arthroscope from the anteromedial portal to look over the lateral dome of the talus. A basket and

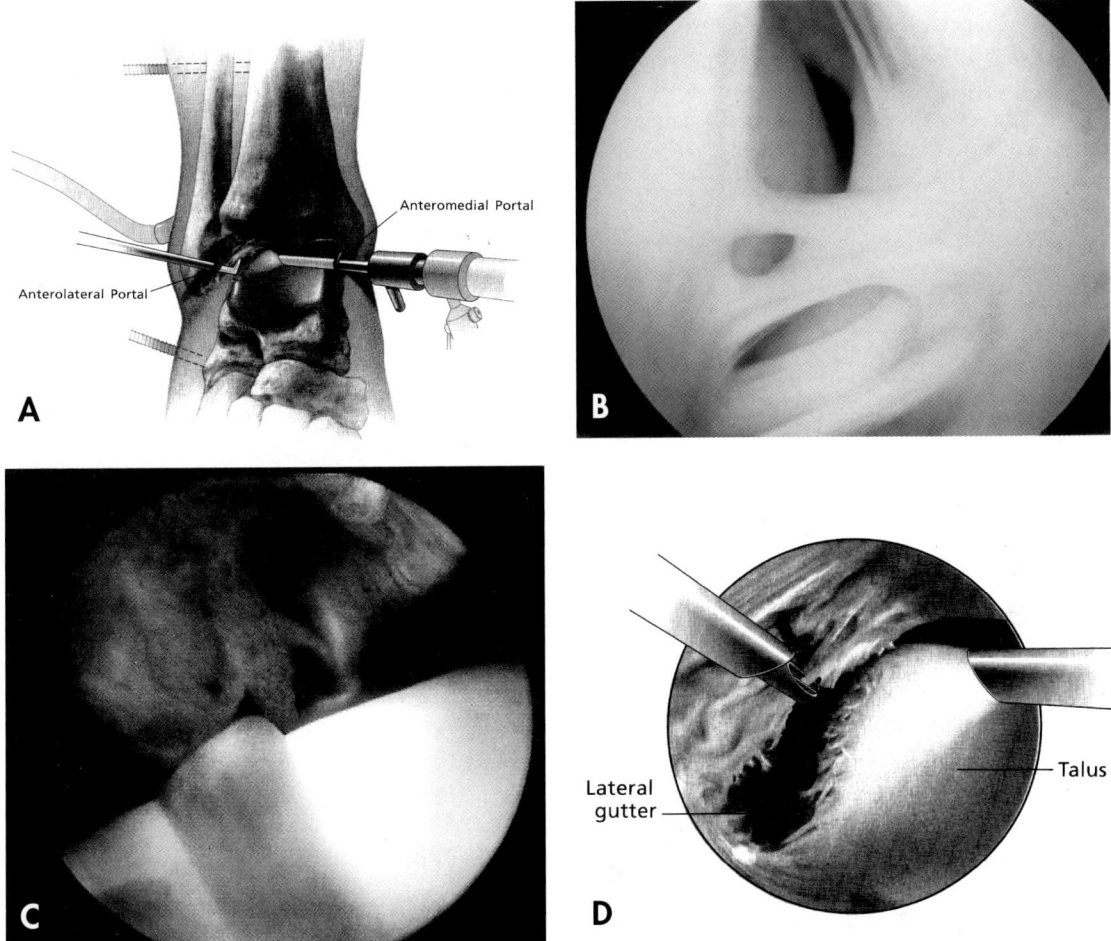

**FIGURE 12**

Anterolateral soft-tissue impingement. **A,** Palpation of scar tissue and fibrotic syndesmotic ligament in a patient with chronic sprain pain. (Reproduced with permission from Jaivin JS, Ferkel RD: Ankle and foot injuries, in Fu FH, Stone DA (eds): *Sports Injuries.* Baltimore, MD, Williams & Wilkins, 1994.) **B,** Arthroscopic view of a left ankle showing multiple scar bands occluding the anterolateral gutter. **C,** Arthroscopic picture in a right ankle showing a scar band abraded against the lateral talar dome and hemorrhagic synovium in the lateral gutter. **D,** Debridement of the anterolateral gutter and scar bands with a small joint full radius shaver in a right ankle. (Reproduced with permission from Jaivin JS, Ferkel RD: Ankle and foot injuries, in Fu FH, Stone DA (eds): *Sports Injuries.* Baltimore, MD, Williams & Wilkins, 1994.)

shaver are used to remove all scar tissue and adhesive bands, inflamed synovium, osteophytes, and loose bodies (Figure 12, *D*). Care must be taken not to excise the ATFL remnant.

Histologic analysis of patients with soft-tissue impingement reveals moderate synovial hyperplasia with subsynovial capillary proliferation in virtually all cases. In some instances, patients also have hyaline cartilage degenerative change and fibrosis consistent with a chronic inflammatory process, but ligamentous tissue generally is not seen on histologic analysis.

### Postoperative Treatment

Each wound is closed with one nonabsorbable suture, and the patient is placed in a posterior splint in neutral position for 1 week. The splint is then discarded after the suture is removed, and a compression stocking and supportive brace are applied. Weightbearing is started at 1 week, and physical therapy usually is started at 2½ to 3 weeks after surgery. Patients can return to full activity, including sports, in approximately 4 to 6 weeks, after completing all the goals of rehabilitation.

## *Results*

Over the last 16 years, more than 180 patients with pain in the anterolateral gutter following an inversion stress injury have been treated. Results initially were analyzed in a smaller group with longer follow-up.[73,74] Eighty-four percent of these patients had excellent and good results. In subsequent follow-up studies, similar results have been obtained. In addition, Liu and associates,[75] Martin and associates,[76] Meislin and associates,[77] DeBerardino and associates,[78] and Ogilvie-Harris and associates[79] have reported similar outcomes in treating this problem.

## SYNDESMOTIC IMPINGEMENT

The inferior tibiofibular ligament is intimately involved with dorsiflexion and plantarflexion of the ankle. The mode of action in the inferior tibiofibular joint depends on the shape of the trochlear surface of the talus. The width of the trochlear surface is smaller posteriorly (2.5 cm) than anteriorly (3.0 cm). Therefore, if the medial and lateral surfaces of the talar body are to be held tightly, the intermalleolar space must vary within certain limits; it must be smallest during plantarflexion and greatest during dorsiflexion.[80]

During plantarflexion of the ankle, the malleoli are approximated actively as the lateral malleolus is pulled inferiorly and rotated medially. Conversely, during dorsiflexion of the ankle, the lateral malleolus moves away from the medial malleolus and is pulled slightly superiorly as the fibula is rotated.[61,81]

Injuries to the syndesmosis are among the most serious that occur to the ankle. Unfortunately, the incidence of these injuries has been underestimated in the past, particularly after an inversion mechanism. In a recent West Point study, 96 cadets suffered ankle sprains. At 6 months, all subjects had returned to full activity, but 40% had residual symptoms. The factor most predictive of residual symptoms was a syndesmosis sprain, regardless of grade.[69] During an acute ankle sprain, if the talus inverts and the tibia rotates, stress is applied across the syndesmosis and a syndesmotic tear occurs. Syndesmotic sprains have been estimated to occur in as many as 10% of all ankle injuries, and tend to be most common in collision sports such as ice hockey, football, and soccer. Syndesmotic sprains may involve any or all of the following structures: the AITF; the posterior inferior tibiofibular ligament (PITF), including its distal and deep components; the transverse ligament; and the interosseous membrane.

## *Clinical Presentation*

On physical examination, patients have extreme tenderness along the syndesmosis and more proximally on the interosseous membrane. A positive squeeze test is usually seen with this injury, as is a positive external rotation stress test.[80,82] Bassett and associates[83] found syndesmotic impingement occurring with a separate distal fascicle of the AITF. After a tear of the ATFL, laxity occurs in the ankle, and the anterolateral talar dome extrudes anteriorly with dorsiflexion, leading to soft-tissue impingement. They did an anatomic study and found the fascicle to be present in 10 of 11 cadavers.[83] I also have seen a separate fascicle of the AITF causing impingement, but I believe that this is traumatically induced rather than a normal variant that may be seen in patients without associated instability.

## *Arthroscopic Appearance*

Syndesmotic impingement is not always seen as an isolated entity. It can also be associated with anterior or posterior impingement. At arthroscopy, the inflamed synovium envelopes the AITF, as well as the inferior articulation of the tibia and fibula. In addition, hemorrhagic synovial nodules frequently are seen in the posterolateral corner of the ankle, just lateral to the PITF. This synovitis can involve not only the anterior but also the posterior aspects of the syndesmotic ligament, and sometimes the ligament may be torn or frayed. Associated loose bodies, chondromalacia, and osteophytes also may be noted.

### *Preferred Method*

After a careful arthroscopic evaluation using the 30° and 70° 2.7-mm short video arthroscopes, a full radius 2.9-mm shaver and suction basket are used to debride the AITF, interosseous space, and posterior syndesmotic ligament. Occasionally, the entire intra-articular portion of the AITF is excised to avoid abrading against the anterolateral talar dome. Previous cadaver studies indicate that approximately 20% of this ligament is seen intra-articularly, and no instability has been caused at this joint by resecting this intra-articular portion.

### *Postoperative Treatment*

The postoperative treatment is the same as previously described for anterolateral soft-tissue impingement, but in some cases patients may take somewhat longer to recover.

## POSTERIOR IMPINGEMENT

Posterior impingement usually occurs laterally, but can also occur centrally or medially. It can be seen alone or in combination with anterolateral or syndesmotic impingement. When it occurs laterally, it usually involves the posterior tibiofibular ligament, posterior interosseous space, transverse tibiofibular ligament, and occasionally, the tibial slip (Fig. 13). A hemorrhagic inflamed posterolateral synovial nodule can develop lateral to the posterior tibiofibular ligament and cause symptoms of pain, swelling, and catching. Pain relief occurs with excision of the nodule and debridement of the surrounding synovitis. A more generalized posterolateral impingement also occurs with fibrosis, capsulitis, and synovial swelling along the posterior portions of the ankle.

Posterior impingement can also be caused by hypertrophy or a tear in the PITF, transverse tibiofibular ligament, tibial slip, or pathologic labrum on the posterior ankle joint (Fig. 14). The tibial slip runs between the PITF and posterior talofibular ligament, and can develop tearing or

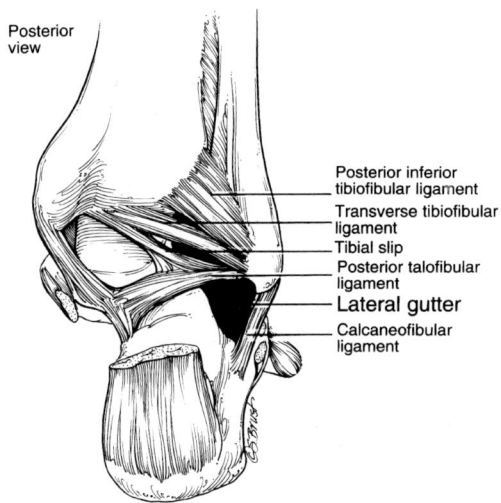

**FIGURE 13**
Posterior impingement sites in the right ankle include the posterior inferior tibiofibular ligament, transverse tibiofibular ligament, and tibial slip. (Reproduced with permission from Ferkel RD, Whipple TL (eds): *Arthroscopic Surgery: The Foot and Ankle*. Philadelphia, PA, Lippincott-Raven, 1996. Susan Brust, medical illustrator.)

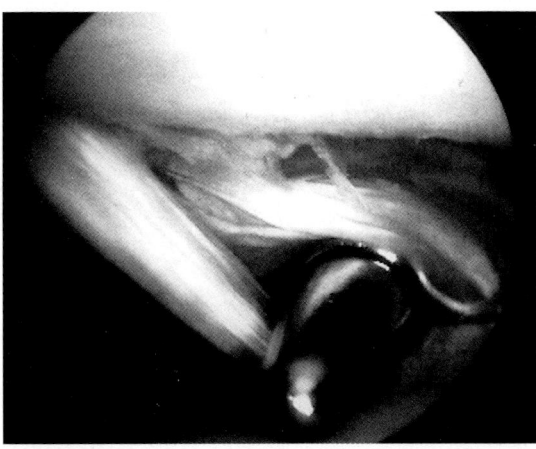

**FIGURE 14**
Tear of the transverse ligament. Note the cannula is between the torn bands of the ligament. This picture is taken while viewing from anteriorly and inserting the cannula from the posterolateral portal.

fibrosis after trauma to the ankle, with subsequent pain and swelling.

Hamilton[84] has described a labrum of the posterior lip or edge of the tibia or posterior "pseudomeniscus," which infrequently can be injured and become hypertrophied or torn, causing significant symptoms.

Diagnosis of posterior impingement problems can be difficult, because radiographs are usually normal or may show calcifications or loose bodies. MRI occasionally may demonstrate hypertrophied ligaments and synovitis or signal change along the posterolateral corner of the ankle.

To diagnose and treat posterior impingement, it is important that the posterior compartment of the ankle is carefully observed through the anterior portals. A distraction device frequently is necessary to permit access to these areas. Treatment usually involves synovectomy with debridement and possible removal of the hypertrophied or torn ligaments. Diagnosis and treatment can also be facilitated by the use of the posterolateral portal, but usually the anterior portals will permit better observation and better access to the pathology.

# LOOSE BODIES

## ETIOLOGY

Loose bodies may be either chondral or osteochondral and may arise from defects in the talus or tibia, osteophytes, or degenerative joint disease.[85] They can occur from either minor or major trauma to the ankle joint. In either situation, an unsuspected chondral or osteochondral lesion may occur, leading to a loose body floating within the joint. Loose bodies can also be seen with osteophytes and, in some cases, both need to be removed at the time of surgery (Fig. 15).

Synovial chondromatosis is associated with multiple loose cartilaginous or osteocartilaginous bodies that form within the ankle joint. This disease is more common in the larger joints, but also can occur in the ankle. In this disease, metaplastic mesenchymal cells in the joint capsule develop into chondroblasts, which produce small clus-

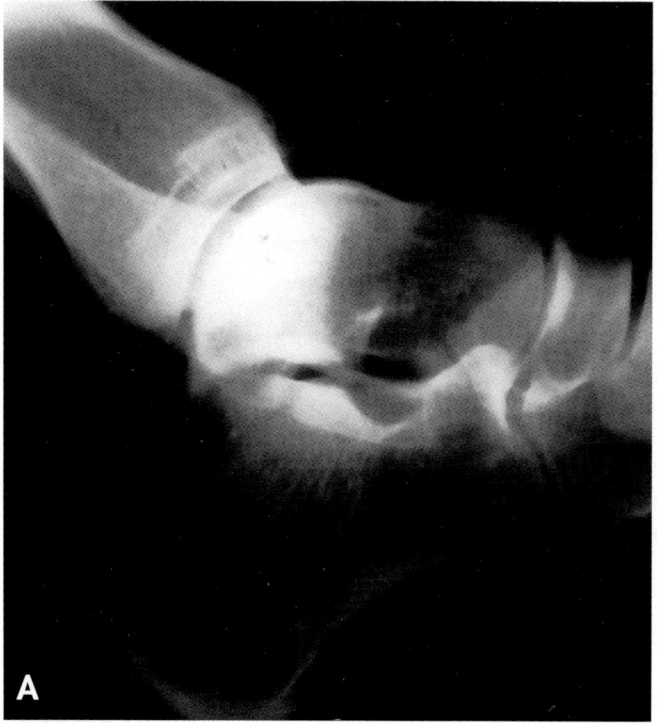
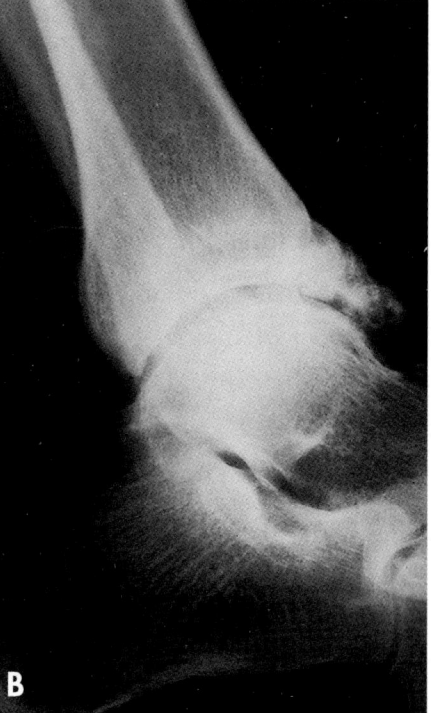

**FIGURE 15**
Osteophytes of the ankle. **A,** Lateral radiograph in 1983 demonstrating minimal osteophyte. **B,** Lateral radiograph in 1999 demonstrating extensive osteophytes anteriorly and some osteophytes posteriorly in the same ankle.

ters of cartilage. These nodules of cartilage can protrude into the joint or break off to form small loose bodies. As the cartilage mass grows, the central portion may become necrotic and calcified. Loose bodies then become visible on routine radiographs (Fig. 16).

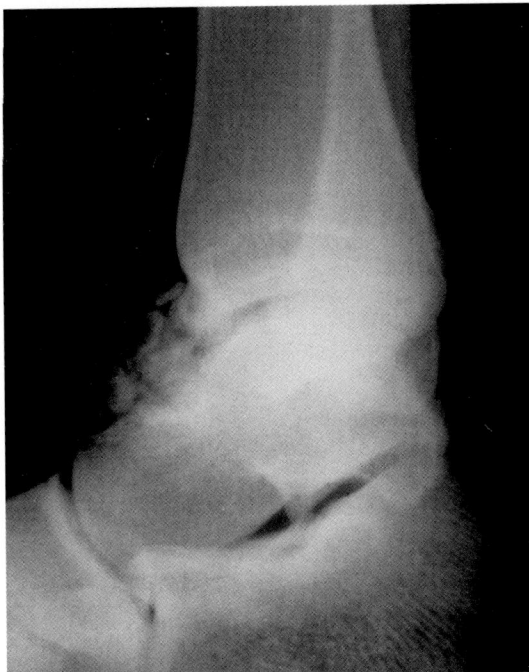

**FIGURE 16**
Lateral radiograph showing multiple loose bodies in a patient with synovial chondromatosis.

## SIGNS AND SYMPTOMS

Loose bodies can cause catching (especially with motion), pain, swelling, and limitation of motion. If the loose body becomes fixed to the synovial lining, symptoms of discomfort within the ankle may resolve. A loose body may grow by proliferation of chondroblasts and osteoblasts, or may shrink because of the action of the chondroclasts and osteoclasts.

The physical examination may not be very revealing, with vague areas of tenderness, possible loss of motion, and catching. Occasionally a loose body can be palpated as it protrudes against the skin. A careful physical examination is very important to rule out extra-articular processes that can cause symptoms similar to those of intra-articular loose bodies. These symptoms include peroneal tendon subluxation, posterior tibial tendon attrition or rupture, tarsal tunnel syndrome, sinus tarsi syndrome, stress fracture, and tendinitis.

## DIAGNOSTIC EVALUATION

Osseous loose bodies are easily seen on plain radiographs, but chondral loose bodies may not be visible on routine studies. An arthrogram, either alone or in conjunction with a CT, usually reveals the loose bodies. Bone scans are rarely helpful with this problem, although MRI resolution has improved enough to help evaluate chondral and osteochondral loose bodies. It is important to discover the origin of the loose bodies, such as a defect of the talar dome, a tibial plafond, or an osteophyte.

Loose bodies can be intra-articular, intracapsular, or extra-articular in location, particularly in the posterior ankle joint compartment. Preoperatively, the location of the loose bodies should be determined on plain radiographs or scans best suited to distinguish between an intra-articular versus an extra-articular or intracapsular abnormality.

## TREATMENT

Generally, loose bodies can be removed arthroscopically, but the procedure can be complicated if multiple loose bodies are present or when appropriate equipment is not available. Posterior loose bodies should be mobilized to the anterior compartment, particularly in patients with ligamentous laxity, so that they can be removed through the anteromedial or anterolateral portals. Not infrequently, posterior loose bodies hide in the posterior recesses of the joint, and this area needs to be carefully checked by palpation. Joint distraction is helpful to see this area.

Anterior joint loose bodies are usually retrieved from the anterior portals. However, when there are multiple loose bodies involved and limited space in which to work, the process can be very tedious and frustrating. Occasionally, it becomes necessary to place the arthroscope in the posterolateral portal and look anteriorly to facilitate loose body removal.

Posterior loose bodies need to be localized and then fixed temporarily with a small needle or guide pin so that they do not move around. Occasionally, when it is not possible to remove the loose bodies through the anterior portals, a grasper can be placed through the posterolateral portal to remove these loose bodies. Special instrumentation has been developed to remove loose bodies arthroscopically from the ankle without damaging the teeth of the smaller flat-head retrieval instrument. After loose bodies are removed, the entire joint surfaces should carefully be evaluated to find the source of the lesion.

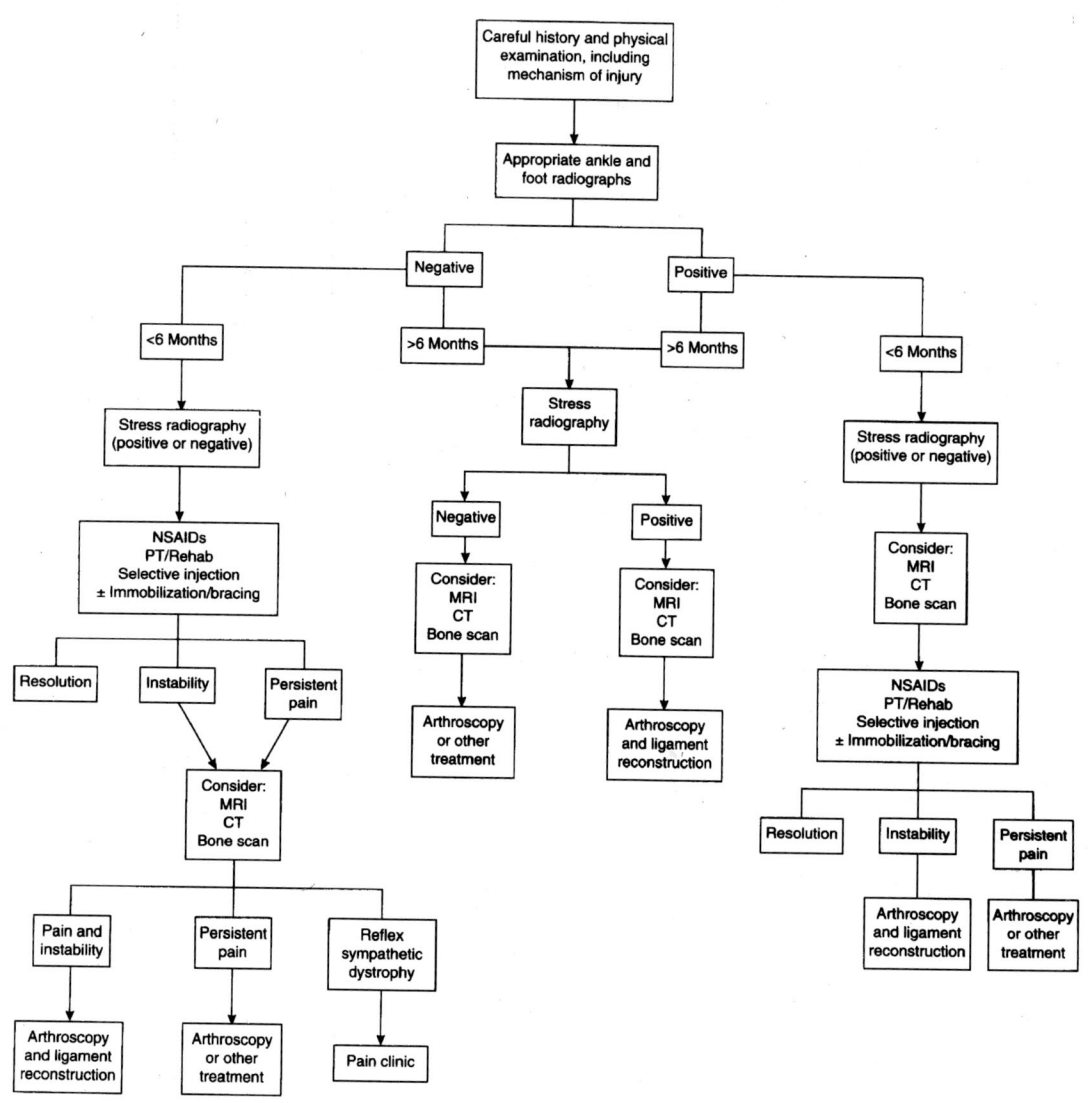

**FIGURE 17**

Algorithm for management of chronic ankle pain. (Reproduced with permission from Stetson WB, Ferkel RD: Ankle arthroscopy: II. Indications and results. *J Am Acad Orthop Surg* 1996;4:26.)

Postoperatively, a bulky compression dressing with a posterior splint is applied. The splint is usually removed in 5 to 7 days after surgery, and exercises are started to regain range of motion. Once range of motion is regained, further strengthening and proprioceptive training are begun.

The clinical results after loose body removal are generally quite good in patients who do not have other associated intra-articular pathology. Results are less predictable when the patient has degenerative or posttraumatic arthritic changes or significant chondral defects.

## CONCLUSION

The challenge of returning an athlete to sporting activity as quickly as possible is an ongoing process. It is critical that the physician communicates well with the patient and his or her parents, trainer, and coach, so that the appropriate treatment is administered while always considering the timetable of the patient's athletic participation. As newer techniques in arthroscopic treatment and rehabilitation of ankle disorders occur, patients will continue to recover more quickly from their nonsurgical or surgical care and be functional in their sports in a much shorter time period. The challenge of treating chronic lateral ankle pain in the athlete is that it requires careful history, physical examination, diagnostic testing, and appropriate treatment. An algorithm (Fig. 17) is also useful to help evaluation and treatment of patients with chronic ankle pain.

## REFERENCES

1. Munro A: *Microgeologie*. Berlin: *Th Billroth* 1856:236.
2. König F: Ueber freie Korper in den Gelenken. *Dtsch Z Chir* 1887;27:90–109.
3. Barth A: Die Entstehung und das Wachsthum der Freien Gelenkkorper. *Arch Klin Chir* 1898;56:507–573.
4. Kappis M: Weitere Beiträge zur traumatisch--mechanischen Entstehung der "spontanen" Knorpelablosungen (sogen Osteochondritis dissecans). *Dtsch Z Chir* 1922;171:13–29.
5. Berndt AL, Harty M: Transchondral fractures (osteochondritis dissecans) of the talus. *J Bone Joint Surg* 1959;41A:988–1020.
6. Campbell CJ, Ranawat CS: Osteochondritis dissecans: The question of etiology. *J Trauma* 1966;6:201–221.
7. Canale ST, Belding RH: Osteochondral lesions of the talus. *J Bone Joint Surg* 1980;62A:97–102.
8. Yvars MF: Osteochondral fractures of the dome of the talus. *Clin Orthop* 1976;114:185–191.
9. Rödén S, Tillegard P, Unander-Scharin L: Osteochondritis dissecans and similar lesions of the talus: Report of fifty-five cases with special reference to etiology and treatment. *Acta Orthop Scand* 1953;23:51–66.
10. Marks KL: Flake fracture of the talus progressing to osteochondritis dissecans. *J Bone Joint Surg* 1952;34B:90–92.
11. Flick AB, Gould N: Osteochondritis dissecans of the talus (transchondral fractures of the talus): Review of the literature and new surgical approach for medial dome lesions. *Foot Ankle* 1985;5:165–185.
12. Pritsch M, Horoshovski H, Farine I: Arthroscopic treatment of osteochondral lesions of the talus. *J Bone Joint Surg* 1986;68A:862–865.
13. Parisien JS: Arthroscopic treatment of osteochondral lesions of the talus. *Am J Sports Med* 1986;14:211–217.
14. Baker CL, Andrews JR, Ryan JB: Arthroscopic treatment of transchondral talar dome fractures. *Arthroscopy* 1986;2:82–87.
15. Pettine KA, Morrey BF: Osteochondral fractures of the talus: A long-term follow-up. *J Bone Joint Surg* 1987;69B:89–92.
16. Van Buecken K, Barrack RL, Alexander AH, Ertl JP: Arthroscopic treatment of transchondral talar dome fractures. *Am J Sports Med* 1989;17:350–356.
17. Anderson IF, Crichton KJ, Grattan-Smith T, Cooper RA, Brazier D: Osteochondral fractures of the dome of the talus. *J Bone Joint Surg* 1989;71A:1143–1152.
18. Bosien WR, Staples OS, Russell SW: Residual disability following acute ankle sprains. *J Bone Joint Surg* 1955;37A:1237–1243.

19. Thompson JP, Loomer RL: Osteochondral lesions of the talus in a sports medicine clinic: A new radiographic technique and surgical approach. *Am J Sports Med* 1984;12:460–463.

20. Blom JM, Strijk SP: Lesions of the trochlea tali: Osteochondral fractures and osteochondritis dissecans of the trochlea tali. *Radiol Clin* (Basel) 1975;44:387–396.

21. Stauffer RN: Intraarticular ankle problems, in Evarts CM: *Surgery of the Musculoskeletal System*. New York, NY, Churchill Livingstone, 1983, pp 8:115–8:142.

22. Yao J, Weis E Jr: Osteochondritis dissecans. *Orthop Rev* 1985;14:190–204.

23. Alexander AH, Barrack RL: Arthroscopic technique in talar dome fractures. *Surgical Rounds for Orthopedics* January 1990, p 27.

24. Zinman C, Wolfson N, Reis ND: Osteochondritis dissecans of the dome of the talus: Computed tomography scanning in diagnosis and follow-up. *J Bone Joint Surg* 1988;70A:1017–1019.

25. Zinman C, Reis ND: Osteochondritis dissecans of the talus: Use of the high-resolution computed tomography scanner. *Acta Orthop Scand* 1982;53:697–700.

26. Ferkel RD, Cheng MS, Applegate GR: Abstract: A new method of radiologic and arthroscopic staging for osteochondral lesions of the talus. Proceedings of the American Academy of Orthopaedic Surgeons 62nd Annual Meeting, Orlando, FL. Rosemont, IL, American Academy of Orthopaedic Surgeons, 1995, p 126.

27. Ferkel RD, Sgaglione NA, Del Pizzo W, Friedman MJ, Snyder SJ, Fox JM: Arthroscopic treatment of osteochondral lesions of the talus: Technique and results. *Orthop Trans* 1990; 14:172–173.

28. Dipaola JD, Nelson DW, Colville MR: Characterizing osteochondral lesions by magnetic resonance imaging. *Arthroscopy* 1991; 7:101–104.

29. Nelson DW, Dipaola J, Colville M, Schmidgall J: Osteochondritis dissecans of the talus and knee: Prospective comparison of MR and arthroscopic classifications. *J Comput Assist Tomogr* 1990; 14:804–808.

30. De Smet AA, Fisher DR, Burnstein MI, Graf BK, Lange RH: Value of MR imaging in staging osteochondral lesions of the talus (osteochondritis dissecans): Results in 14 patients. *Am J Roentgenol* 1990;154:555–558.

31. Lindholm TS, Osterman K, Vankka E: Osteochondritis dissecans of the elbow, ankle, and hip: A comparison survey. *Clin Orthop* 1980; 148:245–253.

32. Alexander AH, Lichtman DM: Surgical treatment of transchondral talar-dome fractures (osteochondritis dissecans): Long-term follow-up. *J Bone Joint Surg* 1980;62A:646–652.

33. O'Farrell TA, Costello BG: Osteochondritis dissecans of the talus: The late results of surgical treatment. *J Bone Joint Surg* 1982;64B:494–497.

34. McCullough CJ, Venugopal V: Osteochondritis dissecans of the talus: The natural history. *Clin Orthop* 1979;144:264–268.

35. Palumbo RC, Kodros SA, Baxter DE: Endoscopic plantar fasciotomy: Indications, techniques, and complications. *Sports Med Arthrosc Rev* 1994; 2:317.

36. Gould N: Technique tips: Footings. *Foot Ankle* 1982;3:184–186.

37. Mukherjee SK, Young AB: Dome fracture of the talus: A report of ten cases. *J Bone Joint Surg* 1973;55B:319–326.

38. Naumetz VA, Schweigel JF: Osteocartilagenous lesions of the talar dome. *J Trauma* 1980; 20:924–927.

39. Ove PN, Bosse MJ, Reinert CM: Excision of posterolateral talar dome lesions through a medial transmalleolar approach. *Foot Ankle* 1989; 9:171–175.

40. Gepstein R, Conforty B, Weiss RE, Hallel T: Closed percutaneous drilling for osteochondritis dissecans of the talus: A report of two cases. *Clin Orthop* 1986;213:197–200.

41. Ferkel RD, Cheng JC: Ankle and subtalar arthroscopy, in Kelikian AS (ed): *Operative Treatment of the Foot and Ankle*. Stamford, CT, Appleton & Lange, 1999, pp 321–350.

42. Ferkel RD: Arthroscopy of the foot and ankle, in Coughlin MJ, Mann RA (eds): *Surgery of the Foot and Ankle*, ed 7. St. Louis, MO, Mosby, 1999, pp 1257–1297.

43. Buckwalter JA, Cruess RL: Healing of the musculoskeletal tissues, in Rockwood CA Jr, Green DP, Bucholz RW (eds): *Fractures in Adults*. Philadelphia, PA, JB Lippincott, 1991, pp 181–222.

44. Buckwalter JA, Mow VC: Cartilage repair in osteoarthritis, in Moskowitz RW, Howell DS, Goldberg VM, Mankin HJ (eds): *Osteoarthritis: Diagnosis and Medical/Surgical Management*, ed 2. Philadelphia, PA, WB Saunders, 1992, pp 71–107.

45. Buckwalter JA, Rosenberg LC, Hunziker EB: Articular cartilage: Composition, structure, response to injury, and methods of facilitating repair, in Ewing JW (ed): *Articular Cartilage and Knee Joint Function: Basic Science and Arthroscopy*. New York, NY, Raven Press, 1990, pp 19–56.

46. Johnson LL: Arthroscopic abrasion arthroplasty: Historical and pathologic perspective. Present status. *Arthroscopy* 1986;2:54–69.

47. Shapiro F, Koide S, Glimcher MJ: Cell origin and differentiation in the repair of full-thickness defects of articular cartilage. *J Bone Joint Surg* 1993;75A:532–553.

48. Kim HK, Moran ME, Salter RB: The potential for regeneration of articular cartilage in defects created by chondral shaving and subchondral abrasion: An experimental investigation in rabbits. *J Bone Joint Surg* 1991;73A:1301–1315.

49. Blevins FT, Steadman JR, Rodrigo JJ, Silliman J: Treatment of articular cartilage defects in athletes: An analysis of functional outcome and lesion appearance. *Orthopedics* 1998;21:761–768.

50. Frenkel SR, Menche DS, Blair B, Watanik NF, Toolan BC, Pitman MI: A comparison of abrasion burr arthroplasty and subchondral drilling in the treatment of full-thickness cartilage lesions in the rabbit. *Trans Orthop Res Soc* 1994;19:483.

51. Mitchell N, Shepard N: The resurfacing of adult rabbit articular cartilage by multiple perforations through the subchondral bone. *J Bone Joint Surg* 1976;58A:230–233.

52. Vangsness CT Jr: Overview of treatment options for arthritis in the active patient. *Clin Sports Med* 1999;18:1–11.

53. O'Driscoll SW: The healing and regeneration of articular cartilage. *J Bone Joint Surg* 1998;80A:1795–1812.

54. Mandelbaum BR, Browne JE, Fu F, et al: Articular cartilage lesions of the knee. *Am J Sports Med* 1998;26:853–861.

55. Borton DC, Peereboom J, Saxby TS: Pigmented villonodular synovitis in the first metatarsophalangeal joint: Arthroscopic treatment of an unusual condition. *Foot Ankle Int* 1997;18:504–505.

56. Brittberg M, Lindahl A, Nilsson A, Ohlsson C, Isaksson O, Peterson L: Treatment of deep cartilage defects in the knee with autologous chondrocyte transplantation. *New Engl J Med* 1994;331:889–895.

57. Minas T, Peterson L: Chondrocyte transplantation. *Op Tech Orthop* 1997;7:323.

58. Jackson DW, Simon TM: Chondrocyte transplantation. *Arthroscopy* 1996;12:732–738.

59. Hangody L, Kish G, Karpati Z, Szerb I, Eberhardt R: Treatment of osteochondritis dissecans of the talus: Use of the mosaicplasty technique. A preliminary report. *Foot Ankle Int* 1997;18:628–634.

60. Yuan HA, Cady RB, DeRosa C: Osteochondritis dissecans of the talus associated with subchondral cysts: Report of three cases. *J Bone Joint Surg* 1979;61A:1249–1251.

61. Ferkel RD, Whipple TL (eds): *Arthroscopic Surgery: The Foot and Ankle*. Philadelphia, PA, Lippincott-Raven, 1996.

62. Brooks SC, Potter BT, Rainey JB: Treatment for partial tears of the lateral ligament of the ankle: A prospective trial. *Br Med J* 1981;282:606–607.

63. McCulloch PG, Holden P, Robson CJ, Rowley DI, Norris SH: The value of mobilisation and non-steroidal anti-inflammatory analgesia in the management of inversion injuries of the ankle. *Br J Clin Pract* 1985;39:69–72.

64. Ruth CJ: The surgical treatment of injuries of the fibular collateral ligaments of the ankle. *J Bone Joint Surg* 1961;43A:229–239.

65. Jackson DW, Ashley RL, Powell JW: Ankle sprains in young athletes: Relation of severity and disability. *Clin Orthop* 1974;101:201–215.

66. Smith RW, Reischl SF: Treatment of ankle sprains in young athletes. *Am J Sports Med* 1986;14:465–471.

67. Anderson ME: Reconstruction of the lateral ligaments of the ankle using the plantaris tendon. *J Bone Joint Surg* 1985;67A:930–934.

68. Freeman MA: Instability of the foot after injuries to the lateral ligament of the ankle. *J Bone Joint Surg* 1965;47B:669–677.

69. Gerber JP, Williams GN, Scoville CR, Arciero RA, Taylor DC: Persistent disability associated with ankle sprains: A prospective examination of an athletic population. *Foot Ankle Int* 1998;19:653–660.

70. Labovitz JM, Schweitzer ME: Occult osseous injuries after ankle sprains: Incidence, location, pattern, and age. *Foot Ankle Int* 1998;19:661–667.

71. Wolin I, Glassman F, Sideman S, Levinthal DH: Internal derangement of the talofibular component of the ankle. *Surg Gynecol Obstet* 1950;91:193–200.

72. Waller JF: Hindfoot and midfoot problems of the runner, in Mack RP (ed): American Academy of Orthopaedic Surgeons *Symposium on the Foot and Leg in Running Sports*. St Louis, MO, CV Mosby, 1982, pp 64–72.

73. Ferkel RD: Soft tissue pathology of the ankle, in McGinty JB, Caspari RB, Jackson RW, Poehling GG (eds): *Operative Arthroscopy*, ed 2. Philadelphia, PA, Lippincott-Raven, 1996, pp 1141–1155.

74. Ferkel RD, Karzel RP, Del Pizzo W, Friedman MJ, Fischer SP: Arthroscopic treatment of anterolateral impingement of the ankle. *Am J Sports Med* 1991;19:440–446.

75. Liu SH, Raskin A, Osti L, Baker C, Jacobson K, Finerman G: Arthroscopic treatment of anterolateral ankle impingement. *Arthroscopy* 1994;10:215–218.

76. Martin DF, Baker CL, Curl WW, Andrews JR, Robie DB, Haas AF: Operative ankle arthroscopy: Long-term followup. *Am J Sports Med* 1989;17:16–23.

77. Meislin RJ, Rose DJ, Parisien JS, Springer S: Arthroscopic treatment of synovial impingement of the ankle. *Am J Sports Med* 1993;21:186–189.

78. DeBerardino TM, Arciero RA, Taylor DC: Arthroscopic treatment of soft-tissue impingement of the ankle in athletes. *Arthroscopy* 1997;13:492–498.

79. Ogilvie-Harris DJ, Gilbart MK, Chorney K: Chronic pain following ankle sprains in athletes: The role of arthroscopic surgery. *Arthroscopy* 1997;13:564–574.

80. Boytim MJ, Fischer DA, Neumann L: Syndesmotic ankle sprains. *Am J Sports Med* 1991;19:294–298.

81. Kapandji IA (ed): *The Physiology of the Joints: Annotated Diagrams of the Mechanics of the Human Joints*, ed 5. Edinburgh, Scotland, Churchill Livingstone, 1987.

82. Hopkinson WJ, St. Pierre P, Ryan JB, Wheeler JH: Syndesmosis sprains of the ankle. *Foot Ankle* 1990;10:325–330.

83. Bassett FH III, Gates HS III, Billys JB, Morris HB, Nikolaou PK: Talar impingement by the anteroinferior tibiofibular ligament: A cause of chronic pain in the ankle after inversion sprain. *J Bone Joint Surg* 1990;72A:55–59.

84. Hamilton WG: Impingement syndromes, in Baxter DE (ed): *The Foot and Ankle in Sport*. St. Louis, MO, Mosby-Year Book, 1995, pp 23–41.

85. Milgram JW: The classification of loose bodies in human joints. *Clin Orthop* 1977;124:282–291.

86. Kumai T, Takakura Y, Higashiyama I, Tamai S: Arthroscopic drilling for the treatment of osteochondral lesions of the talus. *J Bone Joint Surg* 1999;81A:1229–1235.

87. Frank A, Cohen P, Beaufils P, Lamare J: Arthroscopic treatment of osteochondral lesions of the talar dome. *Arthroscopy* 1989;5:57–61.

88. Chin TW, Mitra AK, Lim GH, Tan SK, Tay BK: Arthroscopic treatment of osteochondral lesion of the talus. *Ann Acad Med Singapore* 1996;25:236–240.

89. Baker CL Jr, Morales RW: Arthroscopic treatment of transchondral talar dome fractures: A long-term follow-up study. *Arthroscopy* 1999;15:197–202.

90. Kelberine F, Frank A: Arthroscopic treatment of osteochondral lesions of the talar dome: A retrospective study of 48 cases. *Arthroscopy* 1999;15:77–84.

# NERVE INJURIES OF THE LATERAL LEG AND ANKLE

VINCENT JAMES SAMMARCO, MD, AND LEW C. SCHON, MD

## INTRODUCTION

Chronic lateral ankle pain resulting from nerve injury can be frustrating for the treating physician and a source of severe disability in the athlete. Relatively minor trauma can instigate a series of events that may end an individual's ability to perform at his or her desired level. Injuries to peripheral nerves around the ankle can cause vague, poorly localized symptoms that often are misdiagnosed, delaying treatment and prolonging the disability. Although most nerve injuries resolve with simple rehabilitation initiated by the coach, trainer, or primary-care physician, chronic problems pose major challenges and often are referred to a specialist for diagnosis and treatment.

The athlete can be subjected to several different types of nerve injury: direct blow, stretch, entrapment, and transection. Direct contusions to the leg and ankles cause focal neurologic damage at the site of impact; twisting injuries to the ankle may result in neurapraxias; and repetitive stretching or compression of the nerve in a subclinical fashion may lead to nerve symptoms, which typically occur over the site of a bony edge, fascial band, or tendon. In addition, muscle herniations, soft-tissue tumors (such as ganglions or lipomas), fracture callus, or local anatomic variations (such as accessory muscles) at times are responsible for persistent nerve symptoms. Chronic lateral ankle pain may also result from a nerve transection secondary to a penetrating injury or surgical intervention, eg, open reduction and internal fixation for fibula fractures, reconstruction for lateral instability, or arthroscopy.

Although athletes may suffer injury to any of the nerves of the foot and ankle, this chapter focuses on lateral ankle pain as a result of injury to the superficial peroneal nerve or the sural nerve. We will examine the neuroanatomy, clinical presentation, diagnostic studies, and results of treatment.

## ANATOMY

### SUPERFICIAL PERONEAL NERVE

Knowledge of the anatomic course of the superficial peroneal nerve is essential for proper examination. The superficial peroneal nerve is one of the two large terminal branches of the common peroneal nerve. The common peroneal nerve courses through the thigh with the tibial nerve and then, at the popliteal fossa, courses laterally past the knee joint. After emerging from underneath the lateral insertion of the biceps, it courses around the neck of the fibula and into the lateral compartment. After passing around the fibula neck, the nerve divides into the superficial peroneal nerve and deep peroneal nerve. The superficial peroneal nerve travels deep to the peroneus longus between the muscle and the fibula and descends within the lateral compartment between the peroneus longus and peroneus brevis muscles. In most lower extremities, the superficial peroneal nerve leaves the crural fascia at an average of 13 cm (range, 3 to 18 cm) proximal to the tip of the lateral malleolus.[1] Approximately 15% of the time, the superficial peroneal nerve crosses through the intermuscular septum into the anterior compartment before piercing the crural fascia. The superficial peroneal nerve branches (in another 15 %), and one branch courses in the anterior compartment and the second remains in the lateral compartment.[1]

It is important to appreciate the variability in the two branches of the superficial peroneal nerve, ie, the medial dorsal cutaneous nerve and the intermediate dorsal cutaneous nerve. These two branches divide 4 to 5 cm after exiting the fascia.[1] In approximately 15% of patients, the intermediate dorsal cutaneous nerve branch exits from the lateral compartment and crosses the fibula within a few centimeters of the ankle joint. This variation makes the nerve particularly vulnerable during lateral ankle surgery.[2] It also has been found that when the superficial peroneal nerve pierces the intermuscular septum and courses in the anterior compartment before exiting the fascia, the likelihood of its chronic entrapment is greater.[1]

Awareness of the distal paths of the medial and intermediate dorsal cutaneous nerves is critical to understanding dorsal foot injuries and their sequelae. The medial dorsal cutaneous nerve branches into the dorsal sensory nerve of the medial hallux with variable innervation to the second toe. There is some cross innervation with the deep peroneal nerve to provide sensation in the first web space, but this first web space is innervated primarily by the deep peroneal nerve. At the level of the midtarsus, the medial dorsal cutaneous nerve crosses over the deep peroneal nerve, usually in the region of the bases of the first and second metatarsals and the junction of the medial and middle cuneiforms. When nerve injury occurs at this location, the etiology is usually a direct blow or iatrogenic injury from retraction or inadvertent division of the nerve during surgical fixation of an athletic Lisfranc subluxation or dislocation.

The intermediate dorsal cutaneous nerve branches distally to provide innervation to the dorsal third and fourth web spaces and the dorsal aspect of the third and fourth toes. More proximally, the intermediate dorsal cutaneous nerve courses over the anterolateral shoulder of the talus by the ankle joint; this location sometimes becomes a site of pain secondary to the nerve rubbing or snapping over the talus or its overlying extensor tendons. Anastomoses between branches of the superficial peroneal nerve are common (nearly 50%) on the dorsum of the foot;[3] such anastomoses also occur between the intermediate and medial dorsal cutaneous nerves and the deep peroneal nerve, and between the intermediate dorsal cutaneous nerve and the sural nerve.[3,4] In approximately 20% of patients, the superficial peroneal nerve also sends a motor branch to the extensor digitorum brevis; this is useful information when using electromyography studies to distinguish between lesions of the deep and superficial peroneal nerves.[5–7]

## SURAL NERVE

The sural nerve begins as two nerves in the distal thigh and proximal leg: the medial sural nerve and the communicating branch of the peroneal nerve. The medial sural nerve, a branch of the tibial nerve, pierces the fascia between the medial and lateral heads of the gastrocnemius, emerges with a vein from the popliteal fossa, and courses down the central aspect of the leg posteriorly until it reaches the junction of the middle and lower thirds of the leg. At this point, the medial sural nerve typically anastomoses with the communicating branch of the peroneal nerve, which is a division of the common peroneal nerve. The branch arises from the peroneal nerve proximal to the head of the fibula and courses over the lateral head of the gastrocnemius. It joins (or communicates with) the medial sural nerve in the distal third of the leg and is then called the lateral sural nerve. The lateral sural nerve pierces the fascia and becomes superficial as it crosses over the Achilles tendon.[8,9]

As the lateral sural nerve courses distally, its superficial location makes it more vulnerable to injury. It courses in the sulcus between the peroneal tendons and Achilles tendons, branches toward the posterior and lateral aspect of the heel, and often courses over the sinus tarsi distal to the ankle, frequently sending an anastomotic branch into the intermediate dorsal cutaneous nerve. In the foot, the lateral sural nerve, which is often called the lateral dorsal cutaneous nerve, has branches that course over the bases of the fourth and fifth metatarsals; it often innervates the fifth metatarsal and fifth toe and, occasionally, portions of the fourth toe. The lateral sural nerve also supplies the plantar lateral foot underneath the fifth metatarsal. This nerve is vulnerable during exposure for Achilles tendon procedures, calcaneus fractures, peroneal tendon procedures, lateral Lisfranc injuries, fifth metatarsal fractures, and sinus tarsi surgeries.

## GENERAL CLINICAL PRESENTATION

Individuals who sustain an acute stretch, penetration, or direct blow to a nerve typically have a sudden onset of numbness, burning, tingling, or radiating pain at the time of the initial injury. In cases of nerve injury secondary to repetitive microtrauma, the neurologic symptoms are more subtle, and the physician must obtain an appropriate history to determine whether any of these symptoms have been experienced. Patients with this form of nerve dysfunction sometimes will only begin to experience neural symptoms at high levels of activity, with faster paces, longer distance, incline or decline, uneven terrain, or slippery conditions.

In addition to a thorough peripheral neurologic evaluation, clinical examination must entail a standard physical examination of the foot to discover any malalignment, stress fracture, tendon dysfunction, ligamentous instability, or joint restrictions. Each peripheral nerve should be palpated from proximal to distal in an attempt to elicit the point of maximum tenderness. Percussion along each nerve should be performed similarly, in an effort to identify a trigger point for pain. Zones of decreased or abnormal sensitivity should be noted. The patient or clinician should perform maneuvers that stretch the nerve in the attempt to reproduce the symptomatology. A more generalized neurologic examination should include an evaluation of the L4, L5, and S1 nerve roots to rule out a proximal nerve problem. The examination should also include a quick check of a patient's hands for atrophy, weakness, or neurologic deficit, which may indicate a more systemic problem.

When a nerve injury is suspected, it often can be followed clinically until resolution without the need for further tests. In some cases, however, the intensity or duration of symptoms mandates treatment. In such cases, a more aggressive workup of the involved area may include magnetic resonance imaging to rule out any local factors, such as tendon tears, muscle tears, bone or joint irregularities, or space-occupying lesions, that may be responsible for the patient's nerve symptoms. A bone scan can be helpful for determining whether the condition is associated with any bone or joint pathology. Other studies that may be helpful include stress radiographs of the affected joint. The patient may also benefit from a detailed dynamic gait analysis, in which the physician watches the athlete on a treadmill or on a track or field to determine what that athlete is doing when symptoms begin. If an exertional compartment syndrome is suspected, compartment pressure testing before and after exercise is warranted. A pedobarograph can illustrate plantar malalignments that may affect plantar neurologic structures, particularly the tibial nerve and its branches (ie, interdigital neuralgia). To localize the problem, diagnostic anesthetic blocks of joints, tendons, and nerves may be performed. Nerve blocks should begin distally and then advance proximally in an attempt to isolate the problem area.

If the diagnosis still remains in question, nerve conduction studies and electromyography should be performed to evaluate the location and extent of the problem; that is, to identify whether it is an external compression phenomenon (entrapment) or an intrinsic nerve disorder (axonopathy). Multiple nerve involvement may suggest a peripheral neuropathy or a systemic problem, and more proximal nerve involvement may suggest a radiculopathy.

## NERVE INJURIES WITH ANKLE SPRAINS

### GENERAL
Nerve injury in conjunction with ankle sprains occurs far more often than is expected by treat-

ing physicians (Fig. 1). Most athletes who sustain even mild inversion injuries demonstrate pain and swelling as well as substantial weakness in the musculature surrounding the ankle. Most often, the weakness is caused by pain that inhibits muscle contraction. This weakness, however, can also occur from nerve traction. More severe sprains, in which the ankle mortise is forced well beyond its physiologic range and ligaments are grossly disrupted, often result in major nerve traction injuries that can cause prolonged disability. Approximately 15%[10] of grade 1 and grade 2 ankle sprains[11] demonstrate nerve dysfunction either as weakness in the peroneal musculature or by a subjective instability. Grade 3 sprains are typically associated with more pronounced motor and sensory deficits that may or may not be symptomatic. The three patterns of peripheral nerve injury that can occur in conjunction with an ankle sprain are afferent, efferent, or mechanical.

One pattern of dysfunction after ankle sprain is a feeling of continued instability. The patient usually relates a previous inversion injury and complains that the ankle constantly feels as though it will "give way" or cannot be trusted. Physical examination and stress radiography often are normal. Cohen and Cohen[12] first suggested the concept of arthrokinetic reflexes as an important mechanism in controlling the stability and function of joints. This mechanism depends on proprioceptive input from joint receptors and reflexive firing of certain muscle groups. This concept has been extrapolated to the ankle joint and defined as "functional instability"[13-15] when the proprioceptive receptors in the joint capsule and ligaments are injured, disabling the reflex. Konradsen and Ravn[15] supported this theory by measuring reaction time by monitoring motor responses to sudden inversion in 15 patients with "functional" ankle instability and in 15 patients with normal ankle stability. They found that peroneal muscle reaction time was prolonged in patients with instability and hypothesized that partial deafferentation of the reflex loop was responsible for this abnormality. Thus, loss of the afferent proprioceptive information from the injured joint itself was responsible for the patients' symptoms.

Efferent neurologic pathways can also be profoundly affected during severe ankle sprains. The mechanism of injury has not been proven biomechanically; however, there are several theories about how neural damage may occur. It is well documented that the stretching of peripheral nerves in vivo leads to acute and long-term deficits in intraneural circulation[16,17] and can result in irreversible functional deficits.[18] Normally, the peroneal nerve displaces approximately 4 cm during inversion[19] and is protected by a variety of mechanisms that aid in its gliding.[20] When the ankle is inverted beyond its range, the nerve may be stretched beyond its physiologic limit, resulting

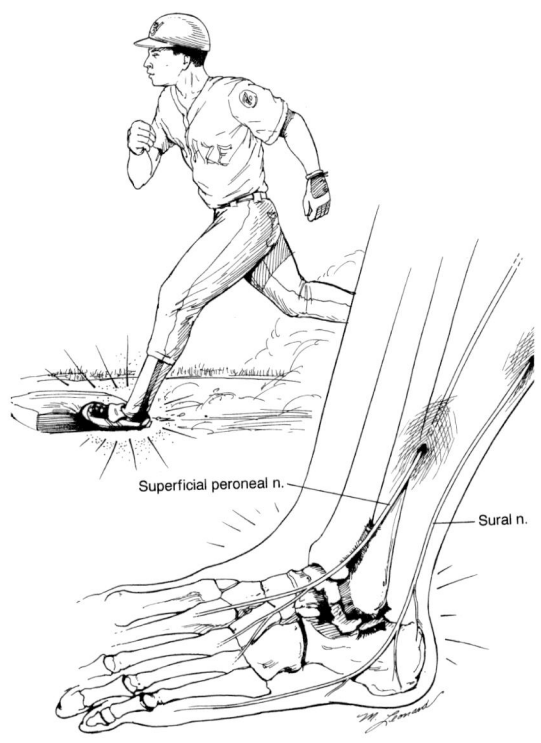

**FIGURE 1**
A lateral ankle sprain may cause a stretch injury of the superficial peroneal nerve or sural nerve. (Reproduced with permission from Schon LC: Nerve entrapment, neuropathy, and nerve dysfunction in athletes. *Orthop Clin North Am* 1994; 25:47-59.)

in a traction injury.[21-23] Several anatomic features may predispose the nerve to injury during inversion injury. When the common peroneal nerve, for example, passes sharply around the fibular neck, a possible tethering point during fast loading exists.[19-22] Anatomic dissections also have elucidated a musculotendinous arch in the peroneus longus muscle that may act as a point of constriction.[19] Any point at which the nerve passes through the crural fascia can act as a site of entrapment, which explains why a nerve with an anomalous course through the intermuscular septum is at higher risk of injury.[24]

Nerve damage from traction injuries (Fig. 2) can occur from direct stretching of the axons.[25] Traction along the path of the nerve may also result in avulsion of vessels and lead to diminished focal nerve blood supply or (rarely) to intraneural hematoma.[26] Typically, traction injuries result in neurapraxia (in which the axons cannot conduct for a short time, but are not disrupted) or axonotmesis (in which the axons are disrupted). Patients with traction injuries have acute paresthesia, dysesthesia, anesthesia, or loss of motor function. As the pain and swelling from the sprained ligaments resolves, persistent discomfort from the injured axons becomes the main focus of the patient's complaints. These symptoms may intensify, as the nerve recovers (reinnervation) and the dysesthesia and paresthesia intensify. Depending on the level of the nerve injury, denervation of the peroneal and anterior compartment musculature can occur. Denervation of the leg may occur as high as the sciatic bifurcation in some ankle sprains, resulting in both posterior tibial nerve and common peroneal nerve signs and symptoms.

A detailed neurologic examination immediately after injury will allow a more accurate assessment than one performed after the ankle swells and becomes weak from disuse. Documenting sensory deficits in a dermatomal pattern provides evidence of neurapraxia or axonotmesis. Motor weakness, especially in the peroneal musculature, may be observed during the few hours after injury. Afterward local pain and swelling make examination difficult for sev-

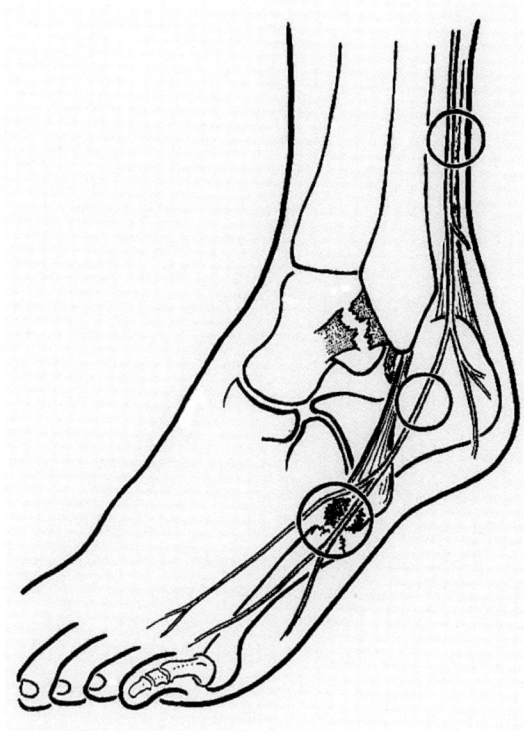

**FIGURE 2**
With an ankle sprain, the sural nerve may be stretched above or below the ankle, as shown in circled areas. With a fifth metatarsal fracture, the sural nerve may be entrapped by callus formation or stretched. (Reproduced with permission from Schon LC, Baxter DE: Heel pain syndrome and entrapment neuropathies about the foot and ankle, in Gould JS (ed): *Operative Foot Surgery*. Philadelphia, PA, WB Saunders, 1994, pp 192-208.)

eral weeks. Whenever the ankle is examined, neurologic assessment should be performed before stressing the ankle ligaments. A stress examination of the ankle ligaments aggravates a patient's discomfort, which conflicts with the subtleties of the neurologic examination.

## TREATMENT
Mild ankle sprains with good peroneal muscle strength (greater than 4/5 or 5/5 at 2 to 3 months) do best with functional rehabilitation. An ankle stirrup and early weightbearing optimize ligament healing, edema resolution, and resolution of mus-

cle atrophy. After 2 or 3 weeks, the patient starts strengthening and range-of-motion exercises in a controlled environment, and activities are increased as proprioception and motor strength improve. Complete resolution of the sprain and any associated neurapraxia should be expected over 2 to 3 months.

More severe sprains with axonotmesis of small branches of the superficial peroneal nerve, common peroneal nerve, or sural nerve can take much longer to resolve. These injuries usually are associated with complete ligamentous disruption of the anterior talofibular ligament and the calcaneofibular ligament, which results in marked swelling and edema. Gentle stress of the ankle will usually demonstrate instability but, as with less severe sprains, pain and swelling will make a good neurologic examination difficult for several weeks. These injuries often are best treated with initial immobilization in a boot walker. Once swelling has subsided and an accurate neurologic examination can be performed, the patient should begin controlled functional rehabilitation that emphasizes early ankle motion while avoiding inversion. Patients with severe peroneal denervation may be safely managed in a boot walker until motor strength returns. If there is a foot drop, a night splint (ankle-foot orthosis) in neutral will prevent continued nerve traction and Achilles tendon contracture that can impede recovery. Until recovery has plateaued, the patient should continue to participate in physical therapy for range of motion and for avoiding atrophy of the uninvolved nerve fascicles.

Sensory denervation after neurapraxia or axonotmesis can be particularly symptomatic. As previously noted, the sensations experienced as the nerve recovers are often painful. There may be excruciating radiating pains of short intensity ("shooters") that are the result of spontaneous discharges from the damaged nerve fibers (ectopic neuralgia). Dysesthesia and hypesthesia in the area of partial denervation are common and uncomfortable. Physical therapy modalities often help control symptoms. Desensitization, whirlpool treatments, and transcutaneous electrical nerve stimulation also may have a beneficial effect.

Medications such as gabapentin (Neurontin), clonazepam hydrochloride (Klonopin), or the tricyclic antidepressants can provide substantial relief for many patients. (This use of these drugs is not approved by the United States Food and Drug Administration, ie, it is off-label.) Low doses of these medications may decrease dysesthesias. The dosage for amitryptiline is usually 10 mg every evening, increasing to 30 to 50 mg/day as the side effects (drowsiness, dry mouth) become more tolerable. Gabapentin can be started at 100 mg every evening and increased to 300 mg/day over the first week. If there is no benefit and if any side effects (such as drowsiness or dizziness) are tolerated, the dose may be increased to 900 mg three times daily if needed. Clonazepam hydrochloride can be started at 0.5 mg orally twice or four times a day. Like other benzodiazepams, clonazepam hydrochloride is sedating and addictive and should be monitored closely.

Because more severe injuries can take 6 months to a year to resolve, narcotic pain medications must be used sparingly. When narcotics are necessary, long-acting agents (such as oxycontin) are less likely to be abused. For patients at risk, a physician-patient narcotic usage contract defines the boundaries of medication used and controls refill requests. Coordination of patient care with a pain management specialist can be helpful for many of these patients.

Most patients with axonotmesis-type injuries recover very slowly at first but make rapid functional gains after the first 6 to 8 weeks. Decreasing frequency of shooters, improved sensation, and increasing peroneal muscle strength are all positive indicators that the injury is resolving. The neurologic examination should be repeated each time the patient is seen and used to chart progress. Axons should grow at the rate of approximately 1 inch per month, and an advancing Tinel's sign along the course of the involved nerve is a good prognostic indication of continued improvement.

If the patient has had no improvement in pain, strength, or sensation after 3 months, the physician should consider electrodiagnostic testing to evaluate for focal demyelination or entrapment. A positive test, severe pain, neurologic deficit, and documented lack of recovery may result from extrinsic nerve compression. These patients may benefit from surgical decompression.

## COMPRESSION NEUROPATHY

Nerve entrapment of the common peroneal nerve, superficial peroneal nerve, deep peroneal nerve, or sural nerve about the ankle is an uncommon sequela of ankle injuries, but has occurred in almost every sport.[10] Players of sports such as soccer and football, in which the lower limbs are subjected to recurrent contusions, are at a higher risk for developing localized entrapment in scar tissue or fracture callus, whereas participants in sports such as dance and distance running are more likely to suffer from entrapment at fascial openings where repetitive motion produces localized microtrauma and scarring. As with other nerve syndromes, diagnosis of compression neuropathy (nerve entrapment) can be extremely difficult and treatment often is delayed.[24, 27]

### ETIOLOGY AND SYMPTOMS

Symptoms usually are insidious in onset.[28,29] There may be a history of antecedent trauma followed by a period of worsening discomfort in the affected dermatome. Common complaints are lateral leg and ankle pain that worsens with exercise. About a third of patients with a compression neuropathy complain of numbness and paresthesia along the course of the nerve,[30] and pain may radiate proximally into the thigh.[31,32] Night pain may or may not be present. Some patients notice a localized swelling or fullness where the nerve pierces the fascia, indicative of a possible muscle herniation compressing the nerve through the fascial defect. Diffuse lateral compartment swelling and firmness with exercise may indicate coexistent exertional compartment syndrome.[33,34] The physician should question the athlete as to whether a specific shoe strap or shin guard exacerbates the condition because the answer may aid in diagnosis. For example, high-top shoes or boots used in specific sports may cause direct compression on the subcutaneous nerves about the ankle.[31,35]

External compression (from shoe wear or other equipment such as shin guards) has been implicated as the cause of neuropathy in the sural nerve, superficial peroneal nerve, and deep peroneal nerve. Because many athletes sacrifice comfort for athletic performance, athletic gear often is worn tightly to increase sensitivity and improve interface with the playing surface. High-level skiers will typically "crank" the buckles on their ski boots to obtain a tight fit, and elite soccer players may buy their shoes so small that they must use petroleum jelly to get their feet inside. Orthotic devices in shoes and wraps or braces may have the same effect as overtightening and can induce nerve compression.

Extrinsic compression of the sural nerve or superficial peroneal nerve may also be due to myositis ossificans,[36] a ganglion,[37] lipoma,[31] or osteochondroma.[38] Callus from fracture of the os calcis[39] or base of the fifth metatarsal[40] has been described as causing entrapment of the sural nerve. Bony entrapment of the superficial peroneal nerve in a fibular callus after fracture of the tibia and fibula can occur.[41]

The superficial peroneal nerve is particularly vulnerable to compression by the fascia of the anterior and lateral compartments as it exits to its subcutaneous position in the distal leg. Lowdon[32] described a nerve that became entrapped as it exited the deep fascia of the lateral compartment, traversing an oblique course through the fascia for more than 1 cm before exiting. In a study of 17 patients (19 legs) with superficial peroneal nerve entrapment, Styf and Morberg[27] defined the "superficial peroneal tunnel" and described a syndrome characterized by lateral leg pain during and after exercise, despite normal intracompartmental pressures. Surgical exploration of these patients revealed a superficial peroneal nerve coursing through a fascial tunnel that was longer than 3 cm. Styf[42] and Styf and Morberg[27] also described three provocative tests that can aid in the diagnosis of distal superficial peroneal nerve entrapment: (1) pressure applied where the nerve emerges from the deep fascia at the anterior intermuscular septum while the patient actively dorsiflexes the ankle; (2) passive stretching of the superficial peroneal nerve by plantarflexing the ankle and inverting the subtalar joint; and (3) percussing the nerve as it is held in the plantarflexed, inverted position. Pain or paresthesia with any of these tests is indicative of superficial peroneal nerve entrapment.

Entrapment of the superficial peroneal nerve also may occur in legs with wide fascial openings where the nerve exits. A large fascial opening may allow muscle or fat to herniate, thus compressing the superficial peroneal nerve at the proximal border of the defect against the fascial edge.[24] As noted previously, nerves that cross through the intermuscular septum into the anterior compartment before exiting the deep fascia are also at higher risk of entrapment.[24] In a series of 21 patients with 24 cases of superficial peroneal nerve entrapment, Styf[24] found that 50% of the cases had herniation of muscle from the lateral compartment where the nerve exits. In 25% of the cases, the superficial peroneal nerve passed through the intermuscular septum before exiting the deep fascia. Styf and Korner[34] also identified an iatrogenic superficial peroneal nerve entrapment at this location after release of the anterior compartment for chronic exertional compartment syndrome. In this circumstance, as the anterior compartment is released, the posterior portion of the compartment retracts posteriorly, collapsing the fascial opening where the nerve exits.

## DIAGNOSIS

Diagnostic studies, such as radiographic studies, magnetic resonance imaging, ultrasound, and electrodiagnostic testing, are often normal. Radiographs may demonstrate a bone or joint abnormality, such as malunited fractures, abundant callus, or osteophytes. Magnetic resonance imaging and ultrasound occasionally may be helpful in identifying soft-tissue lesions in an area of neural entrapment about the ankle.[43] Electrodiagnostic tests are not definitive in ruling out compressive neuropathies because sensory neural action potentials have a high variability (up to 35%) in the legs of normal individuals.[29] Also, because many individuals are asymptomatic at rest, the nerve entrapment and electrophysiologic changes may be observed only with activity.[27] A diagnostic injection of local anesthetic at the site of a suspected entrapment or an adjacent tendon or joint can be very helpful in differentiating pathology. Intracompartmental pressure monitoring can help establish the diagnosis of exertional compartment syndrome. This monitoring is particularly useful when lateral leg pain is present with exercise only.[34,42]

## MANAGEMENT

Compression neuropathy may respond to avoidance of the offending shoe wear or activity. If the symptoms are not controlled with shoe-wear or activity modification, it is unlikely that medication will dramatically improve the patient's complaints. A short trial of nonsteroidal anti-inflammatory medications may prove beneficial for a limited number of patients, and local steroid injection with anesthetic may prove both diagnostic and therapeutic. However, most patients with true extrinsic compression will eventually require surgical release (Fig. 3). Release should not be delayed indefinitely because chronic irritation and entrapment will lead to intrinsic changes in the nerve and perineural fibrosis that may not be reversible with decompression.

Meticulous technique should be used during surgical exposure of the nerve. Often the nerve will be encased in chronic inflammatory tissue or dense scar tissue. Loupe magnification is helpful. The nerve should be approached from a normal section and traced either proximally or distally as it enters the area of entrapment. Care should be taken to perform external neurolysis only, preserving the vas nervosum and leaving much of the perineural fat undisturbed. Extrinsic compression by bony structures requires resection of the prominence. At times, a layer of fascia or fat is interposed between the decompressed nerve and the resected surface. Surgical decompression at a fascial defect requires incision of the fascia for several centimeters proximal to the zone of com-

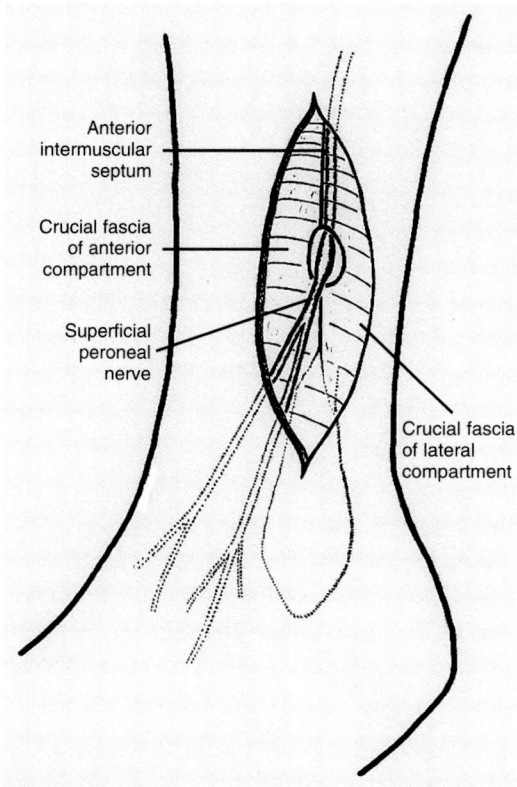

**FIGURE 3**
The superficial peroneal nerve is released where it exits the fascia at the junction of the anterior and lateral compartments. (Reproduced with permission from Schon LC, Baxter DE: Heel pain syndrome and entrapment neuropathies about the foot and ankle, in Gould JS (ed): *Operative Foot Surgery*. Philadelphia, PA, WB Saunders, 1994, pp 192-208.)

pression. Care should be taken to ensure that the nerve is freely mobile after release and that enough fascia has been resected to prevent recurrent entrapment. In the authors' experience, many patients will have dramatic relief after external neurolysis, with 50% to 60% reporting good results within the first few weeks and 80% to 90% reporting benefit by 3 months. Chronic cases of compression with intrinsic nerve damage have an unpredictable recovery.

At times, the symptoms persist despite surgery. This may be due to incomplete release, recurrent fibrosis (adhesive neuralgia), iatrogenic injury, or double-crush phenomenon (two lesions along the course of the same nerve). In the case of incomplete releases, the patient complains that the symptoms are the same as before surgery, that is, they did not change in character after surgery. Repeat electromyographic nerve conduction studies and diagnostic nerve blocks may help in confirming whether the initial surgical site was the point of entrapment. Based on these findings and the physical examination, surgical exploration may include the original surgery site. Care must be taken to completely free the nerve from scar tissue and residual fascial or bony impingement.

Patients suffering from adhesive neuralgia after nerve release are more problematic. Such patients usually have complete resolution of their symptoms in the immediate perioperative period. Some may even return to their normal activity level but, between 2 and 6 months, they experience recurrence of their symptoms. Clinically recurrent fibrosis of the nerve with adhesive neuralgia usually manifests with a tender, thickened surgical scar and neuritic pain induced by motion of the adjacent joint. When nonsurgical modalities such as ultrasound, friction massage, medications, and local steroid injections fail, surgical release may be considered. To minimize recurrent scarring, the nerve should be protected with a barrier graft (fat, muscle, or vein wrap). Overall, patients suffering from adhesive neuralgia do not respond as well to revision surgery as patients whose persistent symptoms are from an incomplete initial release.[44] In the case of double crush from systemic disease or lumbar neuropathy, complete recovery may never occur. At times, it may be necessary to address the other sites of nerve compression to obtain some clinical resolution.

## TRAUMATIC AND IATROGENIC NEUROMAS IN ATHLETES

Neuromas form when both the axons and myelin sheaths of a nerve are severely disrupted. In the foot and ankle, most true neuromas occur as complications of previous surgery (Fig. 4). Ankle ligament reconstruction, surgical treatment of fractures, and ankle arthroscopy are the most common surgical procedures in this population.

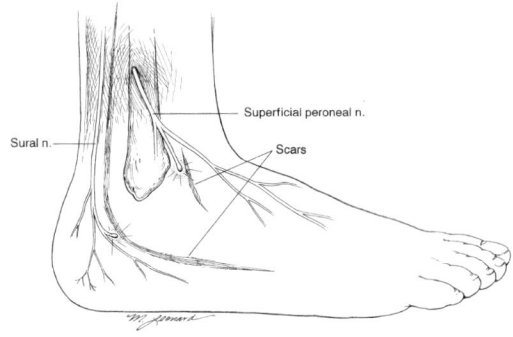

**FIGURE 4**
In surgeries performed in athletes for lateral ankle ligament reconstruction using a peroneal tendon graft (Chrisman-Snook procedure), the sural nerve can be traumatized. Similarly, in an anterolateral approach to the ankle, the superficial peroneal nerve or one of its branches may be injured. (Reproduced with permission from Schon LC: Nerve entrapment, neuropathy, and nerve dysfunction in athletes. *Orthop Clin North Am* 1994;25:47-59.)

These surgeries have a 10% to 15% risk of neuroma formation, either from inadvertent division of a sensory nerve or from excessive retraction during the surgery. Some sports, such as ice hockey and football, place the ankle at high risk of laceration at the upper border of the shoe, and sharp skate blades or metal-tipped cleats can cause substantial damage if the athlete's padding is applied incorrectly. Contusions, crush injury, severe sprains with traction neuropathy, and chronic entrapment may lead to chronic fibrosis that, in extreme cases, becomes a neuroma in continuity.

Histologically, neuromas are disorganized masses of degenerative axonal sprouts and scar tissue that arise from the partially or completely transected nerve.[4] Why some neuromas remain relatively asymptomatic and others are exquisitely tender is unclear. The mechanism by which neuromas generate painful sensation is under investigation. One theory is that mechanical stimulation of the neuroma generates action potentials that may stimulate additional pain signals in dorsal root ganglia (nociceptive neuralgia).[4,45,46] Local accumulations of neuropeptides have been found in experimental neuromas[47] as well as in human sural nerve neuromas.[4] Histamines from infiltrated mast cells and accumulation of substance P and calcitonin gene-related peptide have been found to be abnormally high in these neuromas.[4] Another theory is that there is spontaneous discharge (ectopic neuralgia) that occurs without mechanical stimulation. This discharge may originate from the neuropeptide or neurochemical imbalance in the neuroma, within the proximal nerve, or centrally in the spine. Central nervous system involvement in modulating the impact of these neurochemical responses may help to explain why some patients develop a mild deafferentation phenomenon and others develop a more severe, diffuse hypersensitivity after transection.

In the athlete who previously has undergone a surgical procedure, it is important to differentiate the pain of an incisional neuroma or neuroma in continuity from that of an ongoing mechanical problem. A detailed history is important to define the patient's original presenting complaint. Continued pain as a result of incorrect initial diagnosis or mechanical failure of the surgery should be ruled out in all cases. A patient with postsurgical pain from a neuroma will complain of pain with a character entirely different from that of the preoperative, nonneurologic pain. The postsurgical pain is easily localized by the patient, who will usually complain of symptoms with mechanical irritation of the area (nociceptive neuralgia) from shoe wear or other external stimuli. A neuroma in continuity may be more difficult to diagnose. The primary symptoms are similar to those of traumatic or incisional neuroma, but the history should reveal recurrent injuries, contusion, sprain or entrapment, and not a penetrating event. Symptoms of neuroma in continuity are much less focal than those of incisional neuroma. Burning, tingling, and aching pain are common presenting complaints, and patients may experience dysesthesia and hypesthesia or numbness distal to the site of injury.[48–50] Some patients may experience intense bursts of neuralgia with radiating pain (shooters), which may occur spontaneously (ectopic) or by mechanical irritation (nociceptive).

Palpation and percussion along the course of the affected nerve usually causes radiation of pain both distally and proximally. The entire nerve may be irritable, but a focal area of maximal tenderness usually is present. The examiner should keep in mind that the actual neuroma may not be the patient's main complaint. In the case of a transected nerve, the area of resultant anesthesia can be excruciatingly painful (a syndrome called anesthesia dolorosa). In these cases, percussion of the nerve proximal to the painful area may identify the lesion, although it may not exactly reproduce the symptoms. A deafferentation phenomenon presents with a zone of decreased sensation surrounded by a region of increased sensitivity. The adjacent uninvolved nerves may also become irritable in a deafferentation phenomenon because of effects at the spinal cord level. In such cases, the transected nerve sends signals that lead to augmentation of light touch and pain in adjacent nerves. Such patients are at high risk for developing chronic regional pain syndrome type-II. The physician should carefully examine the patient for signs of vasomotor instability and trophic changes (causalgia) because early recognition leads to early treatment and better outcomes.

Diagnostic injections of local anesthetic can be extremely helpful in localizing the primary focus of pathology. The nerve should be percussed along its course, and the areas of suspected pathology should be noted. If there is more than one suspected area, the distal site should be blocked first. The injection is placed just proximal to the suspected neuroma. After several minutes, the patient is reexamined. If there still is uncertainty about the primary focus, the patient is asked to walk around the office or jog on a treadmill to determine if the symptoms have resolved. This process is repeated until all of the suspected areas have been tested. Some patients will experience dramatic relief with a single injection, which can be impressive in cases of deafferentation pain with adjacent nerve involvement. In such cases, blocking the neuroma often eliminates tenderness of the other nerves. Thus, a single neuroma injection may render asymptomatic a patient who has what appears to be multiple nerve involvement.

If diagnostic injections do not improve symptoms, electrodiagnostic studies may help elucidate a more proximal lesion. Electromyographically guided nerve blocks can be extremely helpful in localizing pathology in an obese patient, in a patient with proximal lesions, or in a patient in whom a conduction deficit has been noted but cannot be reproduced on physical examination. In this procedure, a 25-gauge needle replaces the distal lead in the electromyography apparatus, a slight stimulus is applied, and the needle is manipulated until the patient's symptoms are reproduced. Local anesthetic is then applied through the needle, and the results are noted as above. This usually is done in conjunction with a physiatrist or neurologist, but it is important for the orthopaedist to personally examine the patient immediately before and after the examination to determine its effect.

The treatment for a neuroma and a neuroma in continuity should begin with medication and physical therapy. If an injection of local anesthetic substantially improves the patient's symptoms, a small amount of steroid injected into the area may prove beneficial. The physician should be cautious in the use of steroids because overuse may cause atrophy of the skin and subcutaneous tissues. One steroid injection is indicated, but if this does not provide any lasting relief, additional injections are not advisable. Gabapentin and amitryptiline can provide substantial improvement (uses not approved by the United States Food and Drug Administration). These medications are particularly helpful if multiple nerves are involved through deafferentation or in the setting of vasomotor and trophic changes. Physical therapy is important to maintain range of motion, mobilize edema, and keep muscles as conditioned as possible. Desensitization of the tissues through therapeutic modalities may also have some benefit.

The surgical approach to neuromas includes transection, transection and burial, nerve reanastomosis, and (in extreme cases) peripheral nerve stimulation. For a case of nociceptive neuralgia (mechanical stimulation of the nerve ending), a more proximal transection with or without burial may be sufficient. For a case of ectopic neuralgia (spontaneous neural discharge), anesthesia dolorosa, coexistent chronic regional pain syndrome, or severe deafferentation phenomenon, a more proximal transection and burial may not be sufficient unless there is also a nociceptive component. In patients without a nociceptive component, a transection and burial may increase the symptoms. Such patients represent the minority, and they need to be counseled that the results are less predictable with resection and burial. For severe, recalcitrant cases that have not responded to medications and the aforementioned techniques, two other salvage procedures are available: central (spinal cord) and peripheral nerve stimulation.[51] Results with neurostimulation procedures can be good in terms of relieving overall pain and dysfunction, but a return to athletic activities is not a reasonable expectation.

It is important to discuss with the patient that resolution of symptoms with injection of local anesthetic is no guarantee of complete resolution after transection of the affected nerve. Nerve transection will trigger other local and central responses that may alter the patient's pain and result in new and or different sensations. Also, new neuromas will form at the new proximal level of transection. When multiple nerves are involved after a transection injury, we feel that the risk of additional deafferentation and more global neuralgia in the extremity is increased. Nevertheless, many patients will benefit substantially from transection of the involved nerves proximal to the neuromas. In our practice, we have found that neuromas for which the symptoms are reproduced by mechanical irritation (palpation, percussion, stretch, and ankle motion) and that have good relief with anesthetic injection, will do well with transection of the affected nerve proximal to the neuroma and burial of the end into healthy muscle, or bone. Using these parameters as indicators, success can be as high as 80% to 90%.

Surgical technique should be meticulous and loupe magnification is recommended. The nerve is identified proximal to the neuroma, and dissection is performed cephalad for several centimeters until the surgeon is sure that all involved branches have been identified. At this point, the nerve is sharply transected, and the end placed into healthy muscle tissue or bone proximally. The nerve stump should preferably be at a site that will not be compressed by weightbearing or shoe wear. Care must also be taken to ensure that the nerve is free enough to sit in the muscle tissue or bone without tension, and that motion of the ankle or knee joint does not cause any nerve traction. A 5-0 suture can be used to suture the epineurium to maintain the position of the nerve. Care should be taken to avoid suturing the actual fascicles of the nerve.

## SUMMARY

In summary, chronic lateral ankle pain in the athlete may result from nerve injury. Injuries include traction, compression, contusion, and transection. Most mild cases of acute nerve injury will respond to nonsurgical treatment that is utilized for the primary musculoskeletal ailment. Acute surgical intervention is indicated for transections or for nerve compressions or traction injuries in conjunction with displaced fractures or dislocations. In more chronic injuries the nerve symptoms will often manifest only as the musculoskeletal complaints resolve. When possible, medications should be used in association with injections and physical therapy to facilitate recovery. In recalcitrant cases, nerve surgeries (including nerve releases, nerve releases and barrier procedures, nerve reanastamosis, and nerve transection with or without burial) may be performed. Patients with ectopic neuralgia, deafferenation phenomenon, anesthesia dolorosa, multiple nerve involvements, or chronic regional pain syndrome may do poorly with these conventional approaches and may be candidates for neuromodulation by central or peripheral nerve stimulation.

## REFERENCES

1. Acus RW III, Flanagan JP: Perineural fibrosis of superficial peroneal nerve complicating ankle sprain: A case report. *Foot Ankle* 1991; 11:233–235.

2. Blair JM, Botte MJ: Surgical anatomy of the superficial peroneal nerve in the ankle and foot. *Clin Orthop* 1994;305:229–238.

3. Canovas F, Bonnel F, Kouloumdjian P: The superficial peroneal nerve at the foot: Organisation, surgical applications. *Surg Radiol Anat* 1996;18:241–244.

4. Zochodne DW, Theriault M, Sharkey KA, Cheng C, Sutherland G: Peptides and neuromas: Calcitonin gene-related peptide, substance P, and mast cells in a mechanosensitive human sural neuroma. *Muscle Nerve* 1997;20:875–880.

5. Eastwood DM, Irgau I, Atkins RM: The distal course of the sural nerve and its significance for incisions around the lateral hindfoot. *Foot Ankle* 1992;13:199–202.

6. Reimann R: Accessory peroneal nerves in the human. *Anat Anz* 1984;155:257–267.

7. Zehr EP, Stein RB, Komiyama T: Function of sural nerve reflexes during human walking. *J Physiol (Lond)* 1998;507:305–314.

8. Coert JH, Dellon AL: Clinical implications of the surgical anatomy of the sural nerve. *Plast Reconstr Surg* 1994;94:850–855.

9. Kosinski C: The course, mutual relations and distribution of the cutaneous nerves of the metazonal region of the leg and foot. *J Anat* 1926; 60:274–297.

10. Schon LC: Nerve entrapment, neuropathy, and nerve dysfunction in athletes. *Orthop Clin North Am* 1994;25:47–59.

11. Clanton TO, Schon LC: Athletic injuries to the soft tissues of the foot and ankle, in Mann RA, Coughlin MJ (eds): *Surgery of the Foot and Ankle,* ed 6. St. Louis, MO, Mosby-Year Book, 1993, pp 1095–1224.

12. Cohen LA, Cohen ML: Arthrokinetic reflex of the knee. *Am J Physiol* 1956;184:433–437.

13. Freeman MA, Dean MR, Hanham IW: The etiology and prevention of functional instability of the foot. *J Bone Joint Surg* 1965;47B:678–685.

14. Freeman MA: Instability of the foot after injuries to the lateral ligament of the ankle. *J Bone Joint Surg* 1965;47B:669–677.

15. Konradsen L, Ravn JB: Ankle instability caused by prolonged peroneal reaction time. *Acta Orthop Scand* 1990;61:388–390.

16. Lundborg G: Structure and function of the intraneural microvessels as related to trauma, edema formation, and nerve function. *J Bone Joint Surg* 1975;57A:938–948.

17. Lundborg G, Rydevik B: Effects of stretching the tibial nerve of the rabbit: A preliminary study of the intraneural circulation and the barrier function of the perineurium. *J Bone Joint Surg* 1973;55B:390–401.

18. Kwan MK, Wall EJ, Massie J, Garfin SR: Strain, stress and stretch of peripheral nerve: Rabbit experiments in vitro and in vivo. *Acta Orthop Scand* 1992;63:267–272.

19. Kleinrensink GJ, Stoeckart R, Meulstee J, et al: Lowered motor conduction velocity of the peroneal nerve after inversion trauma. *Med Sci Sports Exerc* 1994;26:877–883.

20. Millesi H, Zoch G, Rath T: The gliding apparatus of peripheral nerve and its clinical significance. *Ann Chir Main Memb Super* 1990;9:87–97.

21. Chapman MW: The use of immediate internal fixation in open fractures. *Orthop Clin North Am* 1980;11:579–591.

22. Meals RA: Peroneal-nerve palsy complicating ankle sprain: Report of two cases and review of the literature. *J Bone Joint Surg* 1977;59A: 966–968.

23. Nitz AJ, Dobner JJ, Kersey D: Nerve injury and grades II and III ankle sprains. *Am J Sports Med* 1985;13:177–182.

24. Styf J: Entrapment of the superficial peroneal nerve: Diagnosis and results of decompression. *J Bone Joint Surg* 1989;71B:131–135.

25. Haftek J: Stretch injury of peripheral nerve: Acute effects of stretching on rabbit nerve. *J Bone Joint Surg* 1970;52B:354–365.

26. Nobel W: Peroneal palsy due to hematoma in the common peroneal nerve sheath after distal torsional fractures and inversion ankle sprains. *J Bone Joint Surg* 1966;48A:1484–1495.

27. Styf J, Morberg P: The superficial peroneal tunnel syndrome: Results of treatment by decompression. *J Bone Joint Surg* 1997;79B:801–803.

28. McAuliffe TB, Fiddian NJ, Browett JP: Entrapment neuropathy of the superficial peroneal nerve: A bilateral case. *J Bone Joint Surg* 1985;67B:62–63.

29. Sridhara CR, Izzo KL: Terminal sensory branches of the superficial peroneal nerve: An entrapment syndrome. *Arch Phys Med Rehabil* 1985; 66:789–791.

30. Schon LC, Baxter DE: Neuropathies of the foot and ankle in athletes. *Clin Sports Med* 1990; 9:489–509.

31. Banerjee T, Koons DD: Superficial peroneal nerve entrapment: Report of two cases. *J Neurosurg* 1981;55:991–992.

32. Lowdon IM: Superficial peroneal nerve entrapment: A case report. *J Bone Joint Surg* 1985: 67B:58–59.

33. Garfin S, Mubarak SJ, Owen CA: Exertional anterolateral-compartment syndrome: Case report with fascial defect, muscle herniation, and superficial peroneal-nerve entrapment. *J Bone Joint Surg* 1977;59A:404–405.

34. Styf JR, Korner LM: Chronic anterior-compartment syndrome of the leg: Results of treatment by fasciotomy. *J Bone Joint Surg* 1986; 68A:1338–1347.

35. Lindenbaum BL: Ski boot compression syndrome. *Clin Orthop* 1979;140:109–110.

36. Husson JL, Blouet JM, Masse A: Entrapment syndrome of the superficial posterior sural aponeurosis. *Int Orthop* 1987;11:245–248.

37. Pringle RM, Protheroe K, Mukherjee SK: Entrapment neuropathy of the sural nerve. *J Bone Joint Surg* 1974;56B:465–468.

38. Montgomery PQ, Goddard NJ, Kemp HB: Solitary osteochondroma causing sural nerve entrapment neuropathy. *J R Soc Med* 1989; 82:761.

39. Miller SD: Sural nerve injury and entrapment. *Foot Ankle Clin* 1998;3:461–471.

40. Gould N, Trevino S: Sural nerve entrapment by avulsion fracture of the base of the fifth metatarsal bone. *Foot Ankle* 1981;2:153–155.

41. Mino DE, Hughes EC Jr: Bony entrapment of the superficial peroneal nerve. *Clin Orthop* 1984; 185:203–206.

42. Styf J: Chronic exercise-induced pain in the anterior aspect of the lower leg: An overview of diagnosis. *Sports Med* 1989;7:331–339.

43. Daghino W, Pasquali M, Faletti C: Superficial peroneal nerve entrapment in a young athlete: The diagnostic contribution of magnetic resonance imaging. *J Foot Ankle Surg* 1997; 36:170–172.

44. Skalley TC, Schon LC, Hinton RY, Myerson MS: Clinical results following revision tibial nerve release. *Foot Ankle Int* 1994;15:360–367.

45. Wall PD, Devor M: Sensory afferent impulses originate from dorsal root ganglia as well as from the periphery in normal and nerve injured rats. *Pain* 1983;17:321–339.

46. Wall PD, Gutnick M: Ongoing activity in peripheral nerves: The physiology and pharmacology of impulses originating from a neuroma. *Exp Neurol* 1974;43:580–593.

47. Zochodne DW, Allison JA, Ho W, Ho LT, Hargreaves K, Sharkey KA: Evidence for CGRP accumulation and activity in experimental neuromas. *Am J Physiol* 1995;268:H584–H590.

48. Kenzora JE: Sensory nerve neuromas: Leading to failed foot surgery. *Foot Ankle* 1986;7:110–117.

49. Lidor C, Hall RL, Nunley JA: Centrocentral anastomosis with autologous nerve graft treatment of foot and ankle neuromas. *Foot Ankle Int* 1996; 17:85–88.

50. Mann RA, Baxter DE: Diseases of the nerves, in Mann RA, Coughlin MJ (eds): *Surgery of the Foot and Ankle,* ed 6. St. Louis, MO, Mosby-Year Book Inc, 1993, pp 543–573.

51. Schon LC, Easley ME: Chronic pain, in Myerson MS (ed): *Foot and Ankle Disorders.* London, England, WB Saunders, 1999.

# INDEX

*Page numbers in **bold italics** refer to figures or figure legends.*

## A

Achilles tendon, 19, ***27***
Acute osteochondral lesions of the talus (OLT)
   repair, 51, ***51***
Adhesive neuralgia, 79
Algorithms
   chronic ankle pain management, 66
Analgesics, 76
Anatomy
   ankle mortise, 6–7
   interosseus ligament, ***12***
   lateral gutter, 59, ***59***
   peroneal tendons, ***17***
   subtalar joint, 21–22, ***22***, 28, ***37, 39, 40***
   superficial peroneal nerve, 71–72
   sural nerve, 72–73
   syndesmosis ligaments, 11, ***11***
   tibiofibular ligaments, ***12***
   variations in, and ankle sprains, 6–9
Anesthesia dolorosa, 82
Ankle mortise, 6–7, 8, ***8***
Ankle sprains
   anatomic variations and, 6–9
   anterolateral impingement of the ankle, 58–62
   classification of, 3–4
   diagnosis, 4–5
   nerve injuries and, 73–77, ***74***
   peroneal tendon injuries, 16–19
   rehabilitation phases, 5–6
   repairs, 9–11
   syndesmosis injuries, 11–16
   treatment and rehabilitation, 5–6, 75–76
Anterior drawer test, 4, ***5***
Anterior process of the calcaneus, 24–25, ***25***
   fracture repair, 25
Anterior talofibular ligament (ATF), ***22***
   reconstruction of, 9, ***10***

Anterior tibiofibular syndesmosis ligament, ***12***
Anterolateral impingement of the ankle, 58–62
Anti-inflammatory drugs, 19, 59, 78, 81
Anticonvulsant drugs, 76, 81
Antidepressant drugs, 76
Arthrofibrosis, 40
Arthrogram, 29
Arthroscopy
   anterolateral impingement of the ankle repair, 60–61, ***61***
   os trigonum excision, 26–27, ***27***
   osteochondral lesions of the talus (OLT) repair, ***51***, 51–54, ***52, 53***
   sinus tarsi syndrome debridement, 34
   subtalar joint instability repair, 29–31, ***30***
   subtalar joint repair, ***38***, 38–40, ***39***
   syndesmotic impingement repair, 63
Arthrotomy, 55
Axonotmesis, 75–77

## B

Bassett's lesion, ***11***
Battle's sign, ***21***
Bifurcate ligament, ***39***
Bone graft, 52, ***53***, 53–54
Bone scan, 2
Braces, 15, 36
Bröstrom procedure, 9–10, 31

## C

Calcaneofibular ligament (CFL), ***22***, 28, ***31***
   reconstruction of, 9
Calcaneonavicular bar
   excision of, 33
Calcaneonavicular coalition, 40
Calcaneus, ***22, 30***
   anterior process, fractures of, 24–25, ***25***
   drilling, 11, ***11***
Calcitonin gene-related peptide, 80
Cannula, 38, 39

Cartilage, 27, 33, 48
Cervical ligament, ***22***, 28, ***31***
Children, talar coalition in, 32, 33
Chondrocyte transplantation, 56
Chrisman-Snook procedure, 10–11, ***11***, 30–31, ***80***
Chronic ankle instability, ***7, 8***, 8–9, ***30***
   repair, 9–11
   subtalar instability and, 30
Chronic ankle pain, algorithm for management of, 66
Chronic diastasis
   repair, 15–16
Chronic lateral ankle pain, 58, 71, 82
Chronic osteochondral lesions of the talus (OLT)
   repair, 51–53, ***52***
Classification
   ankle sprains, 3–4
   lateral process of the talus, fractures of, 23
   osteochondral lesions of the talus (OLT), 46–48, ***47***
   subtalar instability, 28
   syndesmosis injuries, 14
Clinical history, questions for, 1
Coalition. *See* Calcaneonavicular coalition; Talar coalition
Complex regional pain syndrome (CRPS), 2
Complications, 40
   interosseus ligament ossification, 15
   nerve transection, 82
   subtalar joint arthroscopy, 40
   of syndesmosis injuries, 15
Compression neuropathy, 77–79
Computed tomography (CT), 2
   osteochondral lesions of the talus (OLT), 46–48, ***47***
   posteriorly positioned fibula, ***8***
   subtalar joint injuries, 22
   syndesmosis injuries, 13
   talocalcaneal coalition, 33
Cystic lesions, 52–54, ***53***

**D**

Degenerative joint disease, 40
Deltoid ligament laxity, 15–16
Diagnosis
    ankle sprains, 4–5, **5**
    anterior process of the calcaneus, fractures of, 24
    anterolateral impingement of the ankle, 58–59
    complex regional pain syndrome (CRPS), 2
    compression neuropathy, 77–78
    interosseus ligament injuries, 35
    lateral process of the talus, fractures of, 23
    loose bodies, 65, **65**
    nerve injuries, 72
    neurapraxia, 75
    neuroma, 80–81
    os trigonum separation, 26
    osteochondral lesions of the talus (OLT), 27, 43–46
    osteochondral lesions of the tibia, 56
    peroneal tendon injuries, 17–18, 19
    posterior ankle impingement, 36–37
    sinus tarsi syndrome, 34
    subtalar instability, 22, 29, 29–30
    syndesmosis injuries, **12**, 12–14, **13**
    talar coalition, 32–33
    talus, fractures of, 23, 24–25, 27
Dislocations, subtalar joint, 27
Distal peroneus longus tendon injuries, 19
Drilling, 11, **11**, 31, **31**, 51–52, **52**, 53
Dysesthesias, 76

**E**

Ecchymosis, **21**
Ectopic neuralgia, 80, 81–82
Electromyography, 81
Elmslie repair. See Chrisman-Snook procedure
Epinephrine, postsurgical use of, 10
Exercises
    eversion, 6
    proprioception board, **6**
    range of motion, 25
Extensor digitorum brevis, 72
Extensor retinaculum, 9–10, **10**
External rotation stress test, **13**, **14**

**F**

Fibrin glue, 51
Fibula
    drilling, 11, **11**
    Maisonneuve fracture, **12**
    motion of, **7**
    posteriorly positioned, 8, **8**
Fibular groove deepening, 19
Flexor hallucis longus (FHL), 25
Fractures
    anterior process of the calcaneus, **25**
    lateral process of the talus, 23–24
    Maisonneuve fracture, 12, **12**, 13
    metatarsal, **75**
    os trigonum, 26–27
    osteochondral lesions of the talus (OLT), 43–56
    osteochondral lesions of the tibia, 56–57
    posterior process of the talus, 25–26
    subtalar joint, 23–28, 36–37
    treatment and rehabilitation, 23–24, 25

**G**

Grading systems. See Classification
Gutter, lateral, 59, **59**

**H**

Herbert screw, 24
Histamine, 80
History
    osteochondral lesions of the talus (OLT), 43

**I**

Impingement
    anterolateral, 58–62, **61**
    posterior, 36–37
    soft tissue, 57–64, **60**
    subtalar impingement lesion (STIL), 35, **35**
    syndesmotic, 62–63
Inferior extensor retinaculum, **22**, 31, **31**
Intermediate dorsal cutaneous nerve, 72
Interosseus ligament, **12**
Interosseus ligament injuries, 34–36, 40
Interosseus ligament ossification, 15, **16**
Interosseus ligament tear, 12, **35**, 35–36
    treatment and repair, 35–36

Interosseus membrane, 11
    tear, 12, **12**
Interosseus talocalcaneal ligament, 28
Inversion injury, 28

**K**

Kirschner wire, 51, 52

**L**

Larsen procedure, 30, **30**
Lateral process of the talus
    fracture repair, 24
    fractures of, 23–24
Lateral talocalcaneal ligament, **22**, 28, **31**, **39**
Ligament disruption, 3–4
Ligament reattachment, 10
Local anesthetics
    diagnostic use, 2, 59, 81
    postsurgical use, 10
Loose bodies
    diagnosis, 65, **65**
    removal, 65–66

**M**

Magnetic resonance imaging (MRI), 2
    interosseus ligament injuries, 35
    osteochondral lesions of the talus (OLT), 46–48, **49**
    peroneal tendon injuries, **18**
    soft tissue impingement, **60**
    subtalar joint injuries, 22
    syndesmosis injuries, 13, **14**
    talar coalition, 33
    talar cyst, **53**
Maisonneuve fracture, 12, **12**, 13
Medial dorsal cutaneous nerve, 72
Medial heel wedge, 33
Meniscoid lesion, 58
Microfracture pick, **52**
MicroVector drill guide, 51, **52**, 53
Mosaicplasty, 56

**N**

Needles, 38, 39
Nerve decompression, 78–79
Nerve injuries
    adhesive neuralgia, 79
    ankle sprains and, 73–75
    compression neuropathy, 77–79
    neuroma, 79–81
Nerve transection, 81–82
Neural regeneration, 76
Neuralgia, 80–81, 81–82
Neurapraxia, 75–77
Neuromas, 79–81
    neural transection for, 81–82
Nociceptive neuralgia, 82

## O

Occult fractures of the talus, 27–28
Os calcis, 26, **37**
Os trigonum, 25, **26**, 26–27, 36, **37**
    fracture repair, 26–27
Ossification, 32
Osteochondral fractures, 27
Osteochondral grafting, 56
Osteochondral lesions of the talus (OLT), **44**, **49**, **52**
    acute, surgical treatment of, 51, **51**
    anterolateral lesions, 53
    anteromedial lesions, 53
    arthroscopic vs. open repair, 55
    chronic, surgical treatment of, 51–53, **52**
    classification and staging, 46–48, **47**
    cystic lesions, 52–54, **53**
    diagnosis, 27, 46
    etiology, 43–44
    future trends, 55–56
    incidence, 44–45
    mechanism of injury, 45
    nonsurgical treatment, 48–49
    posteromedial lesions, 53–54
    posterolateral lesions, 53
    postoperative care, 54
    repair, 50–54
Osteochondral lesions of the tibia, 56–57
Osteophytes, 64, **64**
Osteotome, **8**

## P

Pain
    chronic lateral ankle pain, 58, 71, 82
    complex regional pain syndrome (CRPS), 2
    management of, 76, 78
    algorithm, 66
    sensory denervation pain, 76
    shooters, 76, 78, 80
Peroneal muscle injuries, 7
Peroneal nerve, **9**
    compression neuropathy of, 77–78
Peroneal tendon injuries, 16–19
    diagnosis, 17–18
    dislocation, **17**, 18
    distal peroneus longus tendon injuries, 19
    repair, 18, 19
    subluxation, 18
    tear, 19
    treatment and rehabilitation, 18–19
Peroneal tendons, **17**
Peroneus brevis tendon, **11**, **18**
    tear, 10–11
Pins, 52
    absorbable, 51, **51**, 54
Plantaris tendon, 31
Posterior ankle impingement, 36–37, **37**
Posterior process of the talus, 25–26, **26**, **37**
Posterior talofibular ligament, **22**
Posterior tibiofibular syndesmosis ligament, **11**, 11, 12, **12**
Posteriorly positioned fibula, 8, **8**
Proprioception board, **6**

## R

Radiography. *See also* Computed tomography (CT); Magnetic resonance imaging (MRI)
    ankle sprain diagnosis, 5
    lateral process of the talus, 23
    osteochondral lesions of the talus (OLT), 46
    peroneal tendon injuries, 18
    subtalar joint, 22, 37
    syndesmosis injuries, 13–14, **14**
    talar coalition, 32–33
    tomographic stress test, 29
Rehabilitation
    ankle sprains, 5–6
    arthroscopic osteochondral lesion repair, 54, 57
    phases of, 5–6
    posterior ankle impingement, 37
    subtalar arthroscopy, 40
    syndesmosis injuries, 15

## S

Screws, 14, **15**, 16, 24, 51
    absorbable, 54
Sensory denervation pain, 76
Shooters, 76, 80
    drug treatment, 76, 78
    surgical treatment, 78
Sickling, 36
Sinus tarsi syndrome
    repair, 34
Soft tissue impingement, 57–64
    repair, 60–61, **61**, 63, 64
Spur debridement, 8–9, **9**
Stenosing tenosynovitis, 27
Stieda's process, 25, **26**, **27**, **39**
Substance P, 80
Subtalar impingement lesion (STIL), 35, **35**
Subtalar joint
    anatomy, 21–22, **22**, 28, **37**, **39**, **40**
    arthroscopic techniques, 29–31, **30**, 37–40, **38**, 38–40
    biomechanics, 21–22
    dislocations, 28
    fractures of, 23–28, 36–37
    interosseus ligament injuries, 34–36
    posterior impingement, 36–37
    radiography, 22, 37
    sinus tarsi syndrome, 34
    tarsal coalition, 32–34
Subtalar joint instability, 22, 28–31, **30**
Subtalar ligament tear, 28
    repair, **30**, 30–31, **31**
Superficial peroneal nerve, **79**
    anatomy, 71–72
    compression neuropathy of, 77
    injury to, **80**
Sural nerve, 72–73
    compression neuropathy of, 77
    injury to, **75**, **80**
Surgical techniques. *See* Techniques
Suture anchors, 10, 11, 18, **19**
Sutures, 11
    absorbable, 9, 19
    nonabsorbable, 16
Syndesmosis injuries
    chronic diastasis, 15–16
    classification, 14
    complications, 15
    diagnosis, **12**, 12–14, **13**
    mechanism of, 12
    radiography, 13–14, **14**
    repair, 14–15, **15**
    treatment and rehabilitation, 14–15
Syndesmosis ligaments, 11, **11**
Syndesmotic impingement, 62–63
Synovial chondromatosis, 65, **65**

## T

Talar coalition, 32–34
    repair, 33–34
Talocalcaneal bar, 33
Talocalcaneal interosseus ligament, **22**, **39**
Talocalcaneal joint, 28
Talocrural arthrosis, **16**
Talofibular ligament, **27**
Talonavicular joint, 27, 28

Talus, **22**, **30**
    cystic lesions of, 52–54, **53**
    drilling, 11, **11**
    lateral process, fractures of, 23–24
    occult fractures of, 27–28
    osteochondral lesions of, 27, 43–56, **51**, 51–54, **52**
    posterior process, fractures of, 25–26, **37**
Tears
    interosseus ligament, 12, 35, **35**
    interosseus membrane, 12
    peroneal tendon, 19
    peroneus brevis tendon, 10–11
    subtalar ligament, 28
    tibiofibular ligament, 63, **63**
Techniques
    arthroscopic techniques
        anterolateral impingement of the ankle repair, 60–61, **61**
        os trigonum excision, 26–27, **27**
        osteochondral lesions of the talus (OLT) repair, **51**, 51–54, **52**, **53**
        sinus tarsi syndrome debridement, 34
        subtalar joint instability repair, 29–31, **30**
        subtalar joint repair, **38**, 38–40, **39**
        syndesmotic impingement repair, 63
    Bröstrom procedure, 9–10, **10**, 31
    calcaneofibular ligament reconstruction, 9–10
    Chrisman-Snook procedure, 10–11, **11**, 30–31

chronic diastasis repair, 15–16
debridement, 34
deltoid ligament repair, 16
drilling, 11, **11**, 31, **31**, 51–52, **52**
Larsen procedure, 30, **30**
ligament repair, subtalar instability, **30**, 30–31
nerve decompression, 78–79
nerve transection, 81–82
os trigonum excision, 26–27
osteochondral lesions of the talus (OLT), 50–54, **51**
    success rate, arthroscopic vs. open, 54–55
peroneal tendon repair, 18–19, **19**
peroneus brevis tendon reattachment, 11, **11**
screw placement, 15, **15**
spur debridement, 8–9, **9**
syndesmosis injury repair, 14–15, **15**
triligament reconstruction, 31, **31**
Tests
    anterior drawer test, 4, **5**
    external rotation stress test, 13, **14**
    tomographic stress test, **30**
    varus stress test, 29, **30**
Thomas heel, 33
Tibiofibular ligament tears, 63, **63**
Tibiofibular ligaments, **12**
Tibiofibular synostosis, **16**
Tomographic stress test, 29
Traction injuries, 75
Treatment, nonsurgical
    ankle sprains, 5–6, 75–76
    anterolateral impingement of the ankle, 59
    axonotmesis, 76

fractures, anterior process of the calcaneus, 25
fractures, lateral process of the talus, 23–24
fractures, os trigonum, 26–27
interosseus ligament injuries, 35–36
occult fractures of the talus, 27
os trigonum fractures, 26
osteochondral lesions of the talus (OLT), 48–49, 50, **50**
syndesmosis injuries, 14–15
talar coalition, 33
Triligament reconstruction, 31, **31**
Trocar, 38
Tubercles, 25–26

**U**

UCB orthosis, 33
Ultrasonography, 18

**V**

Varus hindfoot, 7, **7**
Varus stress test, 29, **30**
Varus tibial plafond, 7
"Vest over pants" suture technique, 9–10, **10**, 16

**W**

Weightbearing, 15, 24, 25, 54

**X**

X-rays. *See* Radiography